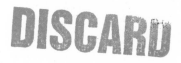

Horse Ailments and Health Care

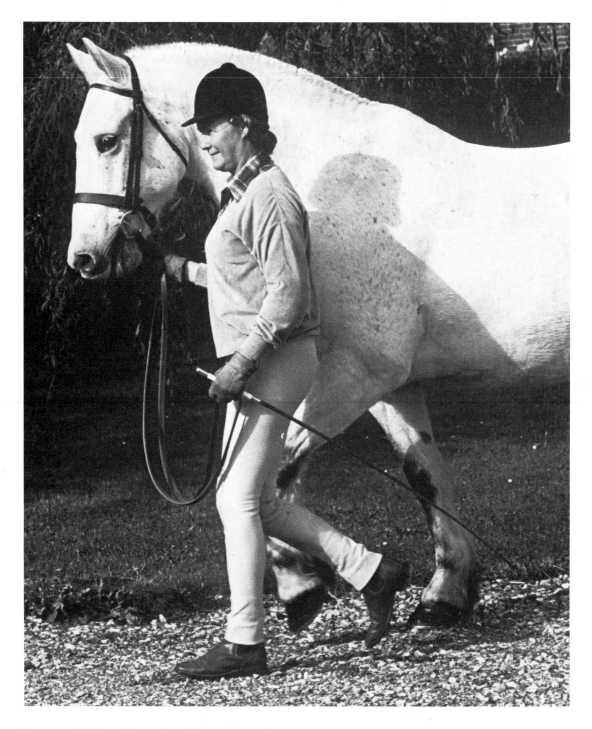

If you are familiar with your horse's appearance when healthy, you will soon learn to recognize when he is not.

A PRACTICAL HORSE GUIDE

Horse Ailments and Health Care

Colin Vogel B.Vet.Med., MRCVS

ARCO PUBLISHING, INC.
NEW YORK

Published by Arco Publishing, Inc.
215 Park Avenue South, New York, N.Y. 10003

First published in Great Britain in 1982
by Ward Lock Limited, London, a Pentos Company.

Library of Congress Cataloging in Publication Data

Vogel, Colin.
  Horse ailments and health care.

  Includes index.
  1. Horses—Diseases. I. Title.
SF951.V63 1982   636.1'0896   82–8684
ISBN 0–668–05632–0   AACR2

Printed in Great Britain

Acknowledgments

I would like to thank my wife, Susan, for ensuring that the text did not attempt to blind the reader with too much science, and also Nicky Savory for deciphering my writing and converting it into a readable typed manuscript.
Colin Vogel.

My thanks are due to L. Roger Falen – Nutritionist, Arizona Feeds, Tucson, Arizona, USA, and to J. R. Overfield, PhD – Central Soya, Decatur, Indiana.
Gillian McCarthy.

Front jacket photograph by David Johnson.
Back jacket photograph by Campbell Goldsmid.
Veterinary equipment for front jacket photograph kindly lent by Arnolds Veterinary Products Ltd, of Reading. Additional equipment kindly lent by Olympic Way, Harrods.

Line diagrams by Hayward Art Group.

Photographs by Marc Henrie, pages 6, 21, 23, 47, 51, 54, 57, 67, 69, 73, 81, 84 and 85; R. M. Ordidge, BVSc, MRCVS, pages 37, 43, 45, 58, 62 and 63; Jane Miller pages 78–79 (taken at Mrs C. P. Blake's Lippen Stud, West Meon, Hampshire; these first appeared in *Birth of a Foal* (1977), J. M. Dent & Sons Ltd); John Elliot, page 2; Egbert van Zon, page 72; Fischer Ultrasound Ltd, page 74.

USA emendations by Matthew Mackay-Smith, DVM, of Delaware Equine Center, Cochranville, Pennsylvania, USA.

Contents

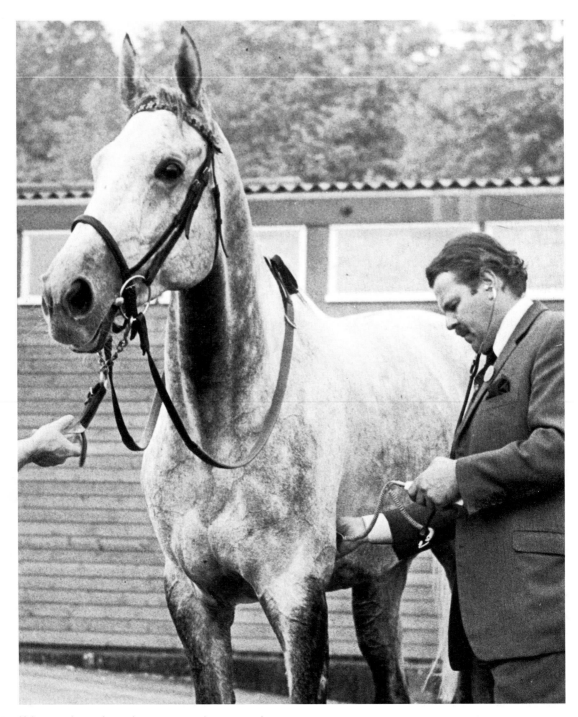

Using an electronic stethoscope, a modern approach to
the old problem of distinguishing slight abnormalities of
sound.

1 Knowing your horse in health

Whatever your reason for buying this book, I ought to make it clear from the outset that this is not a dictionary of symptoms which will enable each horse owner to become his own private veterinary surgeon (veterinarian in USA). Nor is it merely a first aid manual which omits scientific detail as being too complicated for the average reader. My aim is to help you to be able to determine when your horse's health deviates from the normal, and to help you understand the reasoning behind the treatment which you or your veterinary surgeon (veterinarian) may need to carry out in order to restore normal health.

Just as veterinary surgeons (veterinarians) spend half of their lengthy university course studying the normal healthy animal, before even considering what happens in disease, so all horse owners should be familiar with their horse in normal health. If you do not, for example, know how fast a horse usually breathes then you will not be able to tell when he is breathing more quickly than normal.

Any examination for health starts by just looking at the animal. A healthy coat, even in the winter, has a slight sheen to it. The hairs of the coat lie down. When a horse is feeling unwell the muscles in the skin tend to pull the hairs more upright, and this is said to be a 'staring coat'. It is similar to the goose pimples which human beings feel when they are ill with flu etc.

The horse should stand evenly on all four legs. Although horses often rest one leg, especially a hind leg, a healthy horse rests his legs alternately. If a horse rests one particular leg excessively it may indicate that the horse feels some pain when he bears weight on that leg. Horses can, of course, sleep whilst standing up, so they lie down a lot less often than most other animals (including human beings). Horses 'lock' their patella (or kneecap) into position in such a way that the hind legs stay rigid even while the horse nods off. It follows that a horse is unlikely to be so sleepy that he continues lying flat out when you enter the stable. If a horse is unwilling to rise, or lies down again at the very first opportunity, then something is wrong.

Changes can also appear in a horse's behaviour when he is unwell. A horse who is normally very nervous may become quiet and easy to handle, or vice versa. Only if you know your horse's normal behaviour routines in the field or stable can you recognize when that behaviour has changed. Once you have detected a behavioural change you must look closely at the physical signs, in order to discover the reason for the changes.

As you just stand and look at your horse you will also be able to observe his breathing. A resting healthy horse will only take between 8 and 16 breaths per minute. Large horses will tend to be at the lower end of the scale, and smaller ponies will tend to be towards the upper end of the scale. If a horse is breathing faster than 20 times per minute whilst at rest, there is probably something wrong. You should not be able to hear the breathing at all, and it should not be associated with any discharge from the nose, or any coughing.

If for any reason you suspect that your horse might be running a fever, then you should take his temperature before you do anything else which involves handling the horse. This is because when a horse becomes excited in any way its temperature tends to rise. Every stable should possess a clinical thermometer, and you should make sure that you know how to read it. This can be difficult, so practise whilst your horse is healthy and accuracy is not important. A horse's temperature is taken by inserting the thermometer into the horse's rectum and holding it there for about a minute. Always shake the thermometer before use and check that it reads less than 35°C (95°F). Do not take a horse's temperature immediately after he has passed any droppings as you tend then to obtain a false reading. A normal horse's temperature is around 38°C (101°F). If it is above 39°C (102.2°F) then the horse is running a fever.

It is sometimes useful to know how fast your horse's heart is beating. A veterinary surgeon (veterinarian) usually does this by listening to the heart with a stethoscope, but counting a horse's pulse will give just the same information. This again is a procedure which takes a little practice, and so is best perfected on a healthy animal first. (It may help to practise this when your horse has just completed some strenuous exercise. Although the pulse rate will be much increased, the pulse will be stronger and easier to feel.) The pulse is felt by feeling along the inner side of the bottom jaw with the middle two fingers of one hand. You are feeling the blood being forced along a small artery in a rhythmic pulsation.

A healthy horse has a heart rate, and so a pulse rate, of about 40 per minute. As I have already indicated, exercise and excitement can increase this rate up to 100–120 per minute.

Feeling a horse's pulse.

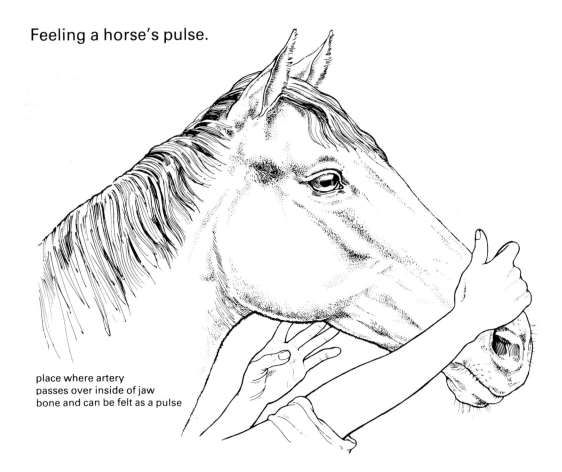

place where artery
passes over inside of jaw
bone and can be felt as a pulse

Although in this chapter, and elsewhere, I am quoting figures for 'a healthy horse' there is much variation. After all, an average is only called an average because there are both higher and lower levels. Although the heart rate and the respiratory rate will vary from horse to horse, one thing remains more or less constant. This is that the horse usually has 3 heart beats for every 1 breath. Any significant variation in this ratio is worth noting. If, for instance, a horse is breathing relatively faster due to pneumonia, then you might well find a heart rate/respiratory rate of only 1:1. If the horse is breathing faster merely because of exercise, then the ratio would stay at around 3:1. It does, however, vary with extremes of temperature and humidity.

You should also be familiar with what your horse feels like. By this I mean that you should know which lumps and bumps are present already, so that you will be able to tell when any small abnormality arises. Even though people groom horses thoroughly, etc. it is amazing how often they are unaware of the presence of small bony lumps such as splints. You should know how firm and straight your horse's tendons feel; how cold or warm his feet normally feel when you enter the stable in the morning. This may all seem to be labouring a point, but being able to answer your veterinary surgeon's (veterinarian's) questions accurately may provide the vital piece of information which enables the correct and speedy diagnosis of an ailment.

One way in which people have often assessed the health or otherwise of a horse is by looking at the membranes around his eyes. Normally these are a salmon pink colour. Beware, however, of the so-called expert who looks at a horse's eye and pronounces that he 'looks a bit anaemic'.

Although these membranes gain their pink colour from the large number of blood vessels which pass through them, the colour of blood does not truly reflect whether a horse is anaemic or not. If a horse has lost a very large volume of blood following an accident then his membranes may well appear pale, but it requires something major like this to happen before our insensitive eyes can really distinguish right from wrong. Similarly it can be difficult to detect obvious signs of jaundice in a horse. Tissues such as fat are usually far more yellow in a healthy horse than in a healthy human being, and it is difficult visually to distinguish between a healthy eye membrane and the eye of a horse suffering from jaundice.

There is one other symptom of normality with which horse riders ought to be familiar. Although we cannot readily hear a horse's breathing at rest, and may well not do so when a horse trots, a horse will always make a noise when breathing at the canter. At this pace breathing and movement are synchronized. The horse breathes out forcibly as the leading leg hits the ground, and this produces a noise. This is not what is meant when people talk of a horse 'making a noise' or 'roaring' at exercise. The term 'roaring' refers to an obvious rasping noise made when the horse breathes in, as well as when it breathes out. If a horse makes a noise when it breathes in at the canter, then this is abnormal.

Once we are sure what a normal healthy horse looks, feels and sounds like, we have a reference point which will help us to know when something is wrong. Firstly, though, there are a number of things we can do to ensure that our horse stays healthy.

2 Routine preventive measures

It is obviously better to take measures to prevent disease rather than to seek to cure an existing ailment. Preventive medicine costs money for professional fees, drugs etc. but it is still cheaper than curing the disease itself. In addition, it may not be possible to return a horse to completely normal health after an illness, due to some permanent damage which has been caused.

Vaccination

Vaccination is a method of preventing illness due to infectious diseases. The infectious organism responsible is injected into the horse in either a dead form or as a live agent which has lost its ability to cause disease symptoms. The horse's body recognizes this foreign antigen (as substances which stimulate the body's natural defences are called) and develops an immunity, or protection, to that specific organism. Usually this protection takes the form of programming certain cells in the blood stream to produce large quantities of a specific neutralizing substance, which is called the antibody. If the horse subsequently comes into contact with a natural infection he will react in the same way, and the protective antibody will neutralize any effects of the disease-producing organism.

In order to understand fully how vaccination programmes work it is necessary to learn a little more about the mechanisms involved. If a dead vaccine is used, i.e. a vaccine containing killed disease organisms, a single injection will be sufficient to programme the 'memory' of the antibody-producing cells, but will not stimulate the production of very large quantities of antibody to circulate in the blood ready for action. This why a dead vaccine always requires two injections. The second injection, which is usually given about four to six weeks after the first, will result in a protective level of antibody being formed and circulated around the blood stream. If a live vaccine is used, the live (but safe) organisms live on in the body for some time and may even reproduce themselves inside the body. They are thus present for a long enough period to both programme the antibody-producing cells and release sufficient antibodies. A single injection is thus sufficient to develop immunity with a live vaccine.

Both live and dead vaccines are usually combined with a substance called an adjuvant. This is a chemical which slightly 'irritates' the tissues around the vaccination site, and generally alerts the body that some sort of response is needed to the vaccine. Adjuvants greatly increase the body's response to a vaccine but they are also responsible for the occasional reactions seen around vaccination sites even with modern vaccines.

TETANUS

Vaccination against tetanus has been practised extensively in horses for many years. Although all animals are susceptible to tetanus, horses are more easily infected than any other domestic animal (although human beings are fairly high up the list as well). Even in treated animals tetanus kills 80% to 90% of affected horses, so prevention is obviously desirable. The disease is caused by a bacterium called Clostridium Tetani. During its life cycle this bacterium forms spores which are so resistant that they can survive for years in soil, etc. Horses are continually taking such spores into their bodies with their food and passing them out in their faeces. In certain conditions where there is a relatively low level of oxygen present but where there is some damaged tissue on which to feed, the spores become active again and the bacteria multiply. Puncture wounds of the foot or into the muscles, and spores lodging in damaged parts of the bowels, are the commonest way in which horses become infected. The bacteria do not make any effort to spread to other parts of the body but they do release a toxin which spreads through the body via the nerves.

The toxin causes tetanic spasms of the muscles controlled by the affected nerves. Commonly the jaw muscles become involved, thus giving rise to the popular name of 'lockjaw'. Death is either due to asphyxiation when the muscles in control of breathing become affected, or due to starvation because the horse is unable to eat or drink. Treatment is aimed at killing the bacteria with antibiotics where possible and simply keeping the horse alive by feeding through a stomach tube, and suspending the horse from slings if it is no longer able to stand etc. Modern muscle-relaxant drugs can help a horse to keep standing, eating and drinking.

It is possible to manufacture an antitoxin against tetanus which does just what its name says; it neutralizes the toxin formed by the already present bacteria. Because it is itself completely foreign to the horse's body, tetanus antitoxin will be destroyed by the cells of the blood within two or three weeks. So antitoxin only provides temporary protection against an existing infection. It is used in treatment of the disease or when an unvaccinated horse sustains an injury.

There should be little cause for the use of tetanus antitoxin because your horses should be vaccinated using tetanus toxoid. This is a dead vaccine which requires two injections separated by approximately four weeks in order to produce long lasting immunity. Booster vaccinations are necessary every one to three years. I must make it clear at this point that no vaccine gives permanent protection. Booster vaccinations are always necessary in order to maintain a high level of antibody circulating in the blood. The 'programming' will last for ever but this response may not be rapid enough to prevent disease if the circulating antibody level has dropped too low.

EQUINE INFLUENZA

Influenza is a very different kind of disease to tetanus. Although it is usually only fatal when affecting young foals, it is extremely infectious to horses of any age. The disease is caused by a virus which affects the respiratory system. Initially the horse may have a fever of about 40°C (104°F) but in many cases this may have returned to normal by the time an owner first notices any symptoms. The horse initially develops a thin clear nasal discharge, which tends to become thicker in character as the disease continues. A cough is present which may persist for as long as three or four weeks. During the height of the disease the horse is obviously unwell, his appetite will be reduced and the horse's performance will be drastically reduced. One serious side effect of the influenza virus which has been noted in past outbreaks is a weakening of the heart and lung tissues. This means that affected horses may need up to six weeks rest after an attack if they are not to end up broken-winded (with scarred lungs) or with a weak heart in a year's time.

The incubation period, which is the period between when the horse comes into contact with the disease and when the first symptoms appear, is usually between three and ten days. Spread of the infection through a susceptible stable yard or group of horses is very rapid; it is the rapid spread of such a debilitating disease coupled with the absence of any drug which will kill the virus which has led to the introduction of vaccination.

Unlike influenza in human beings, which can involve many strains of virus, equine influenza only involves two distinct virus strains (type one and type two). Type one influenza virus is sometimes called the Prague strain, because it was first isolated in that city in 1956. Type two is sometimes called the Miami strain because it was isolated there in 1963. The vaccines commonly available are dead vaccines which contain both viruses. Just as a human being can contract influenza again only a couple of months after an initial outbreak, so immunity following infection with equine influenza is relatively short lived. Although equine influenza vaccines usually carry a recommendation that annual booster vaccinations should be given, there is some evidence that the actual level of protection will start to wane during the second half of this period. It is possible to minimize the effects of any decrease in immunity by vaccination immediately prior to the time of greatest risk. For example, a racehorse should be vaccinated just prior to the start of the racing season, not at the end of it. In some high risk situations it may be advisable to vaccinate against equine influenza every six months or even more frequently.

In Britain there has been since 1981 a move to require compulsory vaccination against equine influenza. This originally applied to all horses entering racecourse premises but has since been extended to other situations where large numbers of horses gather and can be put at risk by the thoughtless horse owner who introduces an already infected horse. The generally accepted definition of a fully vaccinated horse is one which has received two initial vaccinations against equine influenza separated by not less than 21 days and not more than 92 days, and booster vaccinations at intervals of no more than twelve months ever since. Similar vaccination requirements are being introduced in other countries. Vaccination against equine influenza is often combined with tetanus toxoid in a single combined vaccine.

One final word of warning about influenza vaccination. It does not prevent a horse being exposed to infection! Although the majority of vaccinated horses will show no symptoms at all, a small number of vaccinated horses will cough for a couple of days after exposure to the virus. Such symptoms are, however, only slight and of short duration.

RHINOPNEUMONITIS

Although we still commonly refer to the disease of 'rhinopneumonitis', the causal organism is now classified as a herpes virus rather than a rhinopneumonitis virus. When a susceptible pregnant mare becomes infected with rhinopneumonitis she may initially show a slight discharge at the nose, but within seven to ten days she will abort or give birth to a weak premature foal. Such is the infectiousness of the disease that within three or four weeks most of the other pregnant mares which have been in even slight contact with this original mare will also abort. These abortion storms naturally cause economic chaos when they hit a stud farm or even a whole breeding area. The second effect of rhinopneumonitis is to cause a 'snotty nose', which is accompanied by a moist cough and a slight fever.

In the past it has been possible to say that in America the main problem has been abortion caused by the rhinopneumonitis type one virus, and that respiratory symptoms were of little importance. In Britain the main problem has been respiratory symptoms caused by the rhinopneumonitis type two virus, and abortions have been relatively rare. Recently there has been a tendency for the differences to become less clear-cut. In Britain, for instance, the incidence of respiratory disease caused by the so-called 'abortion' type one strain of virus has increased markedly since 1980.

Scientific opinion is slightly uncertain whether immunity against the type one rhinopneumonitis virus will give any cross protection against the type two virus. The vaccines at present available only contain the type one virus. There was a live rhinopneumonitis vaccine available in America for use in preventing rhinopneumonitis abortion. Although very effective, the live virus involved does itself cause an occasional abortion, so these vaccines tend to be used mainly where the incidence of abortion is high. There is also a dead rhinopneumonitis vaccine which is more widely available. The vaccination schedule for this vaccine is rather complicated. Pregnant mares are vaccinated during the fifth, seventh and ninth months of each pregnancy. Non-pregnant mares should be vaccinated on the same schedule as the pregnant mares with which they are in contact as though they were pregnant in May. Other horses should receive two doses separated by three to four weeks with a single dose six months later and annual boosters thereafter. Statistical evidence is still awaited as to the efficacy of dead rhinopneumonitis type one vaccine in dealing with the respiratory problem so often found in Europe.

Worms and worming, and other parasites

Although routine vaccinations are carried out by your veterinary surgeon (veterinarian), routine worming may be carried out by either the horse owner or the veterinary surgeon (veterinarian), depending on how the dose of drug is going to be administered. Some anthelmintics, as the drugs which kill worms are called, are sold already mixed into feed pellets. Unfortunately some horses have an incredible ability to eat a feed and yet leave behind every single pellet containing the worm dose. Other drugs are available in powder or granule form, which can be mixed in with a normal feed. Again, some horses will turn their noses up at the medicated food.

In recent years some anthelmintics have appeared which are made up into a paste form. The appropriate dose is then squeezed out of a syringe onto the back of the horse's tongue, and then swallowed. This method is especially useful for dosing young horses and horses which are not receiving regular supplementary feeding.

In order to ensure that the horse receives the full dose properly, it is often the practice to have such drugs given by the veterinary surgeon (veterinarian) via a stomach tube. This is a painless procedure which involves passing a flexible tube up a horse's nostril and getting the horse to 'swallow' the tube into his oesophagus (gullet), in order that it can be pushed right

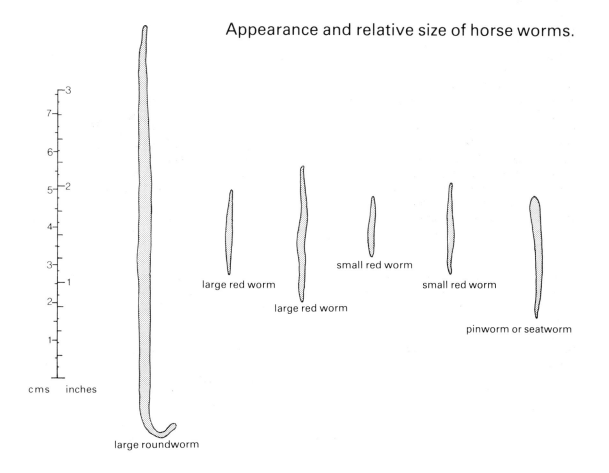

Appearance and relative size of horse worms.

large red worm

large red worm

small red worm

small red worm

pinworm or seatworm

cms inches

large roundworm

down into the stomach. The anthelmintic solution is then poured or pumped directly into the stomach. Although horses may resent the tube being passed through the nasal chambers, they do not feel any discomfort when the fluid is introduced (and appear unaware that it has been given at all).

It is important that every horse owner understands the biology of the worms which can infect horses. Only if you understand what a worm is likely to be doing at any given time, and where it is likely to be found, can you use anthelmintics effectively to prevent too large a worm burden accumulating. It is possible to gain a rough idea of whether a large number of worms are present by examining a horse's faeces under a microscope. The worm eggs present in a known amount of faeces can be counted and expressed as an egg count per gram of faeces but this varies enormously from day to day, and it may not be worthwhile. At the same time the eggs of the two main types of worms, namely ascarids and strongyles, can be readily distinguished. It is also possible to obtain an indication as to the presence of significant numbers of worm larvae, which can, as we will see, cause serious problems. This is done by taking a blood sample and measuring the levels of certain proteins and enzymes in the blood. You should never expect to be able to diagnose the presence or absence of worms by simply looking at the faeces or at the horse's condition.

ASCARIDS

Of the two main types of worm which affect horses, ascarid worms usually only cause problems in young horses. Most foals become infected soon after birth from soil contaminated during the previous year. The ascarid egg has a thick coat which protects it over the winter. In the spring and summer eggs hatch to release infective larvae. Inside the foal the ascarid larvae migrate from the intestines through the lungs until the adult stage is reached back in the intestines when the foal is about three months old. Most adult horses appear to develop an immunity to ascarids, but youngsters may become unthrifty and have digestive upsets.

The migration of large numbers of ascarid larvae through the lungs can cause respiratory symptoms rather similar to a cold, so be on the lookout for worms as a cause of runny noses in young horses.

RED WORMS (BLOOD WORMS)

In older horses the main problems are caused by the so-called 'red worms' (blood worms). The commonest red worm (blood worm), Strongylus vulgaris, has a very complicated life cycle within the horse. The infective larvae of Strongylus vulgaris are consumed whilst the horse is grazing. Within a few days the larvae pass through the wall of the intestines into the actual intestinal arteries. Amazingly the larvae then travel upward through the minute blood vessels until they reach the base of the fan-shaped network of blood vessels which supply the upper part of the small intestine. The immature worms stay three or four months in this site, and inevitably damage the blood vessel walls. Eventually the larvae move on down the arteries until they reach the intestines again. The young adult worms cannot start releasing eggs until they reach sexual maturity after a further six to eight weeks.

Although adult strongyle worms cause some damage to the intestinal wall when they are present in large numbers, the principal damage is caused by the migrating larvae. It is important to note that this is not the stage which can be detected by worm egg counts, nor is it the stage which is treated by routine worming. Larval damage is due to the interruption of the blood supply to the intestines and can result in poor absorbtion of foodstuffs or repeated bouts of colic.

LUNGWORMS

Both horses and donkeys can share another important worm, the lungworm called dictyocaulus arnfieldi. With this worm, larvae picked up from the pasture during the summer months migrate to the lungs where the adult worm remains. Eggs from the lungs pass up to the horse's throat with mucus etc. (a normal defence mechanism which is going on all the time even in horses which are not coughing at all) and are then swallowed. The eggs are thus passed out with the faeces onto the pasture.

Although between 25% and 100% of adult

donkeys may be infested with lungworms, they rarely cause the donkey any problems. In horses, however, the larvae can cause coughing and lung damage. In most horses the larvae never mature to adult worms but just remain in the lungs for a variable length of time. The importance of this fact is that horses infested with lungworms are unlikely to pass any lungworm eggs in their faeces, and worm egg counts are completely unreliable in diagnosing the presence of lungworms. Lungworms should be suspected when:

1　coughing starts in young horses, i.e. under five years old;
2　coughing starts in an animal turned out at grass;
3　there has been any contact, even only indirectly, with a donkey.

WORM PREVENTION

This chapter is headed 'Preventive measures', and worm infestations are definitely something to be avoided. Removal of droppings from the paddocks is an effective but time-consuming way of reducing the number of worm larvae present on the pasture, as is harrowing paddocks to scatter and dry dung in warm weather. Grazing cattle and sheep with the horses will also remove some of the dangerous larvae. The treatment of horses with anthelmintics must not be looked on as an annual or half-yearly chore. After all, such treatment is reducing the number of eggs passed out onto the grazing for future infections, not reducing the number of strongyle larvae causing damage to the intestines at this time. Treatment must be repeated every 4 to 8 weeks if we are to keep worm infestations down to acceptable levels on pastures which are grazed continually by horses.

There is a wide range of anthelmintics available for use in the horse. A drug may be available in one country but not in others. Among the active ingredients commonly found are thibendazole, fenbendazole, dichlorvos, haloxon, (trichlorfon in USA), mebendazole cambendazole, oxfendazole, febantel and pyrantel. Generally speaking these drugs, when used at the recommended dose levels, kill adult worms. They do not affect any migrating larvae that may be present in the body. It follows that if you worm your horse properly, then on the following day there will be no adult worms present in the bowels, and no worm eggs being passed out in the faeces. There will still be migrating larvae present, however, and the time taken between worming and the reappearance of adult egg-laying worms in the bowels will depend on the life cycle of that particular worm. The time taken between a horse picking up new worm eggs from the pasture and these giving rise to adult worms in the bowels is much longer, and is called the prepatent period. For ascarids the prepatent period would be three months, while for strongyles it would be in the region of six months.

Obviously not all drugs are equally effective at killing all the species of worms. Piperazine has been used as an anthelmintic for many years, but it is only really effective against ascarids. Thibendazole is effective against both ascarids and strongyles, but it needs a very much higher dose in order to kill strongyles than is necessary for ascarids. This emphasizes the importance of reading the instructions on the package carefully, and checking with your veterinary surgeon (veterinarian) that you are using the correct drug at the correct dose. Another point to remember is that it may well be false economy to purchase the cheapest anthelmintic you can find. Phenothiazine is sold quite cheaply as an anthelmintic, but it is not effective against ascarids and is quite toxic to horses.

When thibendazole was first discovered it was extremely widely used throughout the world as an equine anthelmintic. Over the years, however, in Britain, America, Canada and Australia cases have been found where strongyles have become resistant to this drug. This has prompted several pharmaceutical companies to develop further drugs from the same molecule, e.g. fenbendazole, oxfendazole, cambendazole, febantel and mebendazole. Unfortunately these new drugs, whilst retaining their own individual advantages as anthelmintics, have inherited this same susceptibility to worm resistance. I mention this because it is pointless to alternate your choice of anthelmintic between members of this group, thinking that you will avoid drug resistance by so doing. The only way to definitely avoid drug resistance with these drugs is to alternate them with a completely different family of drugs, or to use a drug such as pyrantel which has not shown any signs of drug resistance.

I mentioned earlier that most equine anthelmintics do not remove migrating worm larvae from the horse. It is possible to achieve this by using large doses of thibendazole (or some similar compounds such a fenbendazole), usually given by stomach tube. Oxfendazole is claimed to remove a high percentage of migrating strongyle larvae at the normal dose. It is also necessary to take other special measures to kill lungworms in horses, some of which are quite toxic to the horse as well.

Some anthelmintics, e.g. carbon disulphide, dichlorvos and trichlorfon, are also effective against horse bots, which are not worms at all but the larval stage of a fly. Eggs laid on the hairs of the horse's body hatch to larvae, and these larvae migrate through the body before passing out in the faeces. The presence of large numbers of larvae can cause problems, and dosing with such an anthelmintic during the winter months may well be advisable.

Dental care

Just as the presence of large numbers of worms can result in a horse losing weight despite the fact that it is eating well, so tooth problems can result in a horse losing condition. At one extreme a horse's teeth may cause so much pain that it will not chew at all, and so loses condition because it is off its food. At the other extreme the discomfort may only arise when the horse is being ridden in a bridle and being required to react precisely to delicate aids, as in dressage. In between will be the more common case where, because of some discomfort, the horse does not chew its food as thoroughly as it should do. The stomach and bowel contents are not then digested as efficiently as they should be, i.e. you are wasting expensive food.

The horse has six incisor teeth in each jaw for grazing. Then there is a gap (where we place the bit) which may or may not have a small canine tooth on each side in male animals. Finally there are the molar teeth, or cheek teeth, which do the actual chewing. Some horses have a very small 'wolf tooth' immediately in front of the upper molars on one or both sides. Because the horse

Tooth eruption at different ages.

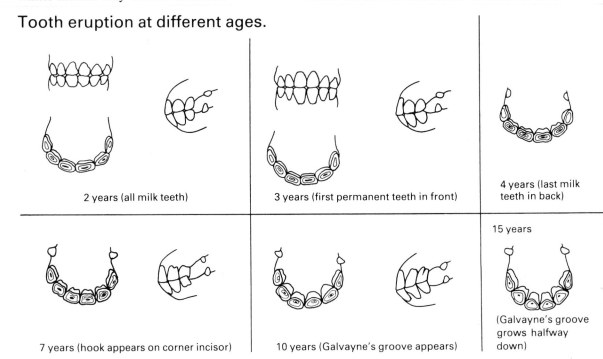

2 years (all milk teeth)

3 years (first permanent teeth in front)

4 years (last milk teeth in back)

7 years (hook appears on corner incisor)

10 years (Galvayne's groove appears)

15 years

(Galvayne's groove grows halfway down)

changes its initial baby incisors for its permanent teeth at regular intervals, it is possible to age a horse fairly precisely up to the age of 8 years old. A foal possesses all its temporary incisor teeth by 9 months old. The first two permanent incisor teeth push out and replace the temporaries at about 2½ years old. These are the centre two teeth of the row of six. At around 3½ years old the adjoining permanent teeth erupt, and at 4½ years old the final two permanent incisor teeth appear. After this stage it is possible to age the horse by examining the amount of wear which has occurred on the biting surfaces of the teeth, but this is a fairly complicated process outside the scope of this book.

The grinding surfaces of a horse's molar teeth are not horizontal, as one might expect. Instead the normal chewing action produces sloping surfaces. The grinding action tends to produce sharp points on the teeth. Usually it is the outside edge of the upper molars and the inside edge of the lower molars which develop these points. The sharp points catch on the tongue and the cheek membranes and cause painful ulcers to form.

These sharp points can be removed from the teeth by a process known as rasping or floating. Firstly your veterinary surgeon (veterinarian) may well insert a gag (piece of equipment which keeps the mouth open) into your horse's mouth in order to prevent the horse closing his upper and lower jaws tightly together. This also enables him to examine the surfaces of the back teeth without any risk of losing a finger! The tooth rasp is then moved backwards and forwards along the edges of the offending teeth

Tooth wear: cross-section of mouth showing tongue and teeth on either side.

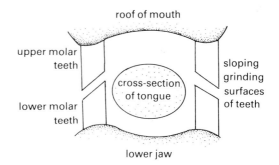

until all sharp points have been removed. It is difficult to make firm rules as to how often this procedure needs to be carried out, but every horse should have its teeth properly checked at least once a year, even if no problems are anticipated.

The small wolf teeth can also cause discomfort. Because of their size these teeth do not have a large root embedded in the jaw bone, but are only embedded in the gums. Pressure from the bit tends to 'rock' these teeth and cause slight pain which prevents the horse responding to the bit as well as he might do. Routine removal of these teeth is often practised in horses which are involved in competition work.

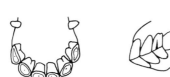

5 years (all permanent teeth)

30 years (Galvayne's groove disappears)

17

Vices

Because treatment of vices such as crib-biting, wind-sucking and weaving is not very successful, prevention must be the aim. Stable vices are primarily due to boredom, so active steps to prevent boredom should be taken. Stabling horses for long periods without any distractions, as can happen in large racing stables, leads to boredom. Horses like to be able to see what is going on in the yard or stable, and to be able to see as much as possible of other horses. Although such vices are not infectious in the sense that, say, equine influenza is, other horses readily copy the habit. For this reason you should think twice about introducing a horse with one of these vices into a yard or stable or barn.

Weaving is when a horse stands (almost as if in a daze) and 'weaves' his head from side to side, in the same way that a lonely child will sit and rock itself. A horse may weave inside the loosebox (box stall) or with his head through the half open stable door.

Crib-biting starts with a horse taking firm hold of some convenient edge in his stable, e.g. the top edge of the stable door, and then grinding his teeth together. This tends to wear away the front edges of the horse's incisor teeth, a point to be looked for when buying a horse. The horse may then learn that if he holds tight with his teeth he can swallow air down into his stomach, and this process seems to be pleasurable or at least gives the horse something to do. Wind-sucking is the final stage, where the horse has learnt to swallow air without needing first to anchor his jaws on a fixed object. Horses suffering from these vices tend not to be good doers (good keepers).

Wood and bark chewing, and eating soil or even dung, are 'vices' which may very occasionally be caused by nutritional deficiencies.

Two different tooth rasps.

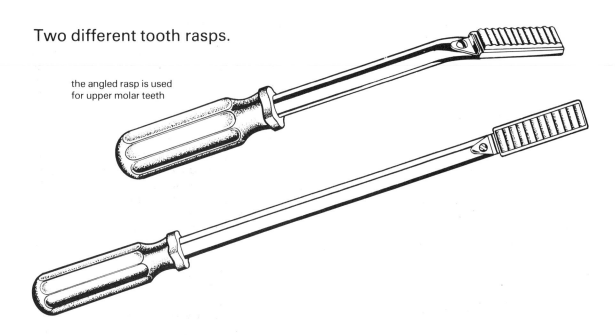

the angled rasp is used for upper molar teeth

3 Calling the vet (veterinarian), and being prepared

Even though you take active steps to prevent your horse having any health problems, sooner or later something will go wrong. Your knowledge of your own horse when he is in normal health will enable you to tell that something is wrong, and that it is time to contact your veterinary surgeon (veterinarian). You should choose the veterinary surgeon (veterinarian) who is going to look after your horse because he or she is interested in and good at working with horses, not because you have heard that they charge the lowest fees in the district or because they just happen to be the nearest one to you. In some countries the professional bodies which regulate the veterinary profession allow specialization, and in these countries the telephone book etc. may list certain veterinary surgeons (veterinarians) as equine practitioners or specialists. In other countries such specialization is frowned upon because it reflects the veterinary surgeon's (veterinarian's) interests and practice rather than any specialist training and qualifications. In these countries, which include Britain, you will often have to rely on word of mouth recommendations as to whether a particular veterinary surgeon's (veterinarian's) practice deals mainly with horses or with hamsters and other small animals etc.

You should make sure that you are familiar with how the veterinary practice is organized, so that you know when is the best time to contact them about arranging a routine visit, and when is the best time to contact them to discuss a particular problem etc. Veterinary surgeons (veterinarians) are quite happy to discuss even minor problems with you, and indeed by doing so may well save you the expense of an unnecessary professional visit. They must, however, be treated like normal human beings! This means that, unless otherwise requested, you should not contact them during the evenings or weekends unless you have an emergency case which needs attention. If you think you have got an emergency, make sure that you state the fact clearly, so that your need for immediate attention is made clear. Veterinary practices (but not necessarily the individual veterinary surgeons (veterinarians) who make up that practice) should have a telephone which is manned 24 hours per day, three hundred and sixty-five days of the year.

It is false economy to delay obtaining professional advice in the hope that the problem will just vanish. An example of this might be severe tendon injuries. Some owners do not present these to the veterinary surgeon (veterinarian) until days or weeks after the damage was sustained. Treatment of such cases should, however, be commenced as soon as possible if it is to have any effect on the course of the illness. Delay means a lost opportunity to influence a case for the better.

One further word of advice about you and your relationship with your veterinary surgeon (veterinarian). Always try to make clear beforehand the problems which you wish to discuss on a particular visit. If the veterinary surgeon (veterinarian) thinks he is only coming to see one horse, he will only allow sufficient time to deal with one horse when he plans his round. If you then expect him to look at three more horses 'while you are here' then three things will happen. Firstly you will annoy the veterinary surgeon (veterinarian) (whether he shows it or not). Secondly you will make him late for all his following appointments, which may include you next time! Thirdly, and most significantly, the discussion of your problems will inevitably be rushed and less detailed than if things had been properly explained in the beginning.

The basic first aid kit

Every stable should possess at least one first aid kit. I say 'at least one' because whenever a horse leaves the yard or stable by horsebox (horse van) or trailer, a first aid kit should go along as well and preferably one should be permanently in the stable. It is no use having the correct bandages etc. for an injury if they are in the tack room at home and the injured horse is out hunting 20 miles (32 km) away.

The first aid kit should include some means of cleaning the wound. Over 90% of all wounds are contaminated with dirt when they occur, and the sooner this dirt and potential for infection is removed, the better. Repair of the wound can wait. A clean wound can be left for an hour or so until a decision is made as to what is the best form of treatment, but a dirty wound is deteriorating all the time. The first aid kit should therefore include some mild disinfectant solution or surgical soap which can be added to the water used for cleaning the wound. Some cotton wool or other swabs, or cotton gauze squares should be available for actually cleaning the wound. Special moist swabs are available which are manufactured for cleaning the skin prior to surgery, and these are ideal for use in the field, where clean water may not be available. These may be obtainable from your veterinary surgeon (veterinarian), or, in the USA, from a surgical supply pharmacy. Clean the wound gently, carefully and thoroughly.

After cleaning, the next stage is to try and prevent any infection becoming established. For this purpose I recommend an antiseptic dusting powder or spray. Some veterinary surgeons (veterinarians) supply their clients with an antibiotic aerosol which is ideal for this purpose. Ointments, however, are not recommended at this stage (despite the fact that many proprietary (ready-made) first aid kits contain them). Although antiseptic powders etc. can be easily washed off later if the wound requires stitching etc., ointments are not so readily removed. A thick application of the traditional 'green oils' may well make you feel that you have done something for your horse, but it may prevent a veterinary surgeon (veterinarian) from being able to suture (stitch) a wound which really ought to be stitched.

Wounds which are bleeding will clot much sooner if firm pressure is applied to them. Gamgee tissue is the best form of padding to use, as it combines the protective qualities of cotton wool with a gauze covering, which eliminates the problem of 'fluff' sticking to the wound. It is possible to obtain packets of specially

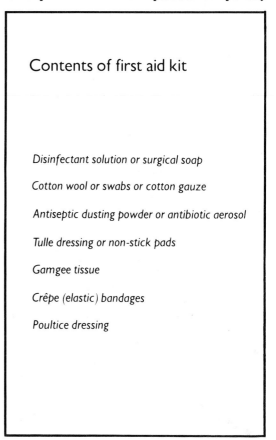

Contents of first aid kit

Disinfectant solution or surgical soap

Cotton wool or swabs or cotton gauze

Antiseptic dusting powder or antibiotic aerosol

Tulle dressing or non-stick pads

Gamgee tissue

Crêpe (elastic) bandages

Poultice dressing

impregnated tulle (non-stick pads in USA) which can be placed directly over a wound and will never stick in place no matter how much oozing occurs. This prevents the frustration of restarting the bleeding each time you change the dressing. The padding can be held in place by crepe (elastic) bandages (ordinary cotton or gauze bandages have no elasticity and are of no use in bandaging horses). Self-adherent stretch bandages are very good but more expensive. The aim is to apply the bandage sufficiently tightly to keep the dressing on, but not so tight that you impede the circulation in any way. There are also various elastic net dressings on the market for holding dressings in place. The disadvantage of these is that often they do not provide sufficient pressure on the wound to stop bleeding. Keeping dressings on a horse's knee or hock has always presented special difficulties. A recent development has resulted in the availability of special lycra dressings which fit firmly over the affected area and hold the dressing in place.

Finally no first aid kit would be complete without some form of poultice dressing. The traditional kaolin poultice is now available in sealed foil envelopes which are much easier to handle than a whole tin of poultice and heat up to the required temperature within minutes rather than hours. In Britain there are also 'Animalintex' poultices. These consist of a dry dressing which requires soaking in water before use. All these poultices can be used cold or ice cold in the case of tendon injuries, or hot where the aim is to draw out the infection, e.g. when a horse cuts his sole on a flint or other sharp object out riding.

A pair of round-ended scissors and a thermometer may also be useful.

There are on the market some ready made first aid kits which have the advantage of keeping the items together in one container. Anyone considering purchasing one of these can look at the contents and compare them with my suggestions in order to make sure that they are adequate.

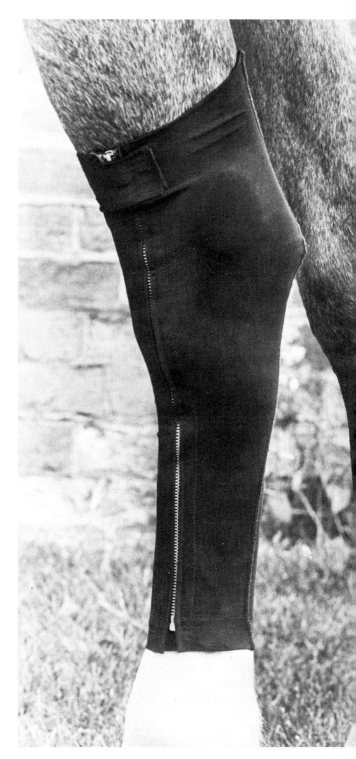

Lycra dressing, the 'Pressage' stretch contour bandage, available in different sizes and for various parts of the leg, fastening with a zipper and 'Velcro'.

21

Wound care

Wound healing in the horse depends very much on the site of the particular wound. Wounds which lie over a part of the body which moves freely, e.g. the knee or the stifle, do not heal well. The aim is always to treat wounds in such a way that they will heal by 'first intention', which means that the two skin edges on either side of the wound stick to each other over the cut. Unfortunately wounds left to themselves tend to heal by 'second intention', which means that the two skin edges do not stick together, and healing is delayed until sufficient new tissue is formed to fill the gap between the cut surfaces and then for new skin to grow over the gap.

The tissue which fills the gap in a wound healing by second intention healing is called granulation tissue. Its name stems from the fact that it has a pink granular appearance. Unfortunately the horse has an unusual tendency to form too much granulation tissue. Instead of merely filling the gap between the broken skin edges, this tissue can grow so exuberantly that it forms a raised lump of 'proud flesh'. Without treatment this proud flesh may never heal or go away, and it is the unfortunate outcome of many neglected wounds. It is obviously wiser whenever possible to aim at first intention healing of wounds, rather than to rely on the slower, and cosmetically less desirable, second intention healing.

Successful wound healing depends on:
The amount of skin lost.
The firmness with which the skin is applied to the underlying tissues.
The amount of movement of the affected part.
The physical condition of the wound, whether wet or dry.
The amount of infection present.

Cuts above the level of the knee and hock generally heal better than those lower down the legs, where the continual movement of tendons etc. tends to inhibit healing.

The problem the horse owner often faces is 'does this wound require veterinary attention or not?' As a general rule I would say that in wounds where:

there is spurting bleeding which may come from an artery

there is bleeding which does not stop after being pressure bandaged for 5 to 10 minutes

there is a cut more than 2.5 cm/1 in long through the whole thickness of the skin

there are puncture wounds in a horse which has not been vaccinated against tetanus

then a veterinary surgeon (veterinarian) should always be called. In deciding whether to suture (stitch) a wound or not, he will obviously be influenced by factors such as the knowledge that where the natural pull of the skin pulls the two cut surfaces together, as with a vertical cut on a horse's leg, the sutured (stitched) cut will heal much better than where the cut surfaces are pulled apart, as with a horizontal cut. It may well be possible to suture small cuts using only a local anaesthetic injected around the wound, with possibly a sedative to quieten the horse.

Wound healing.

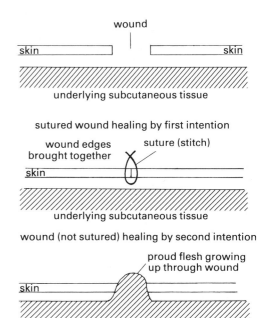

wound

skin   skin

underlying subcutaneous tissue

sutured wound healing by first intention

wound edges   suture (stitch)
brought together

skin

underlying subcutaneous tissue

wound (not sutured) healing by second intention

proud flesh growing
up through wound

skin

underlying subcutaneous tissue

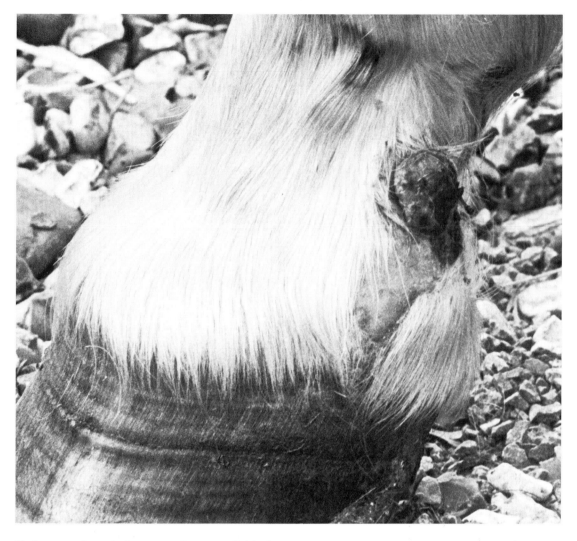

Proud flesh at a pastern wound.

Unfortunately sedatives are often unreliable in their effect on already excited horses, and horses with wounds tend to be excited. Because the veterinary surgeon (veterinarian) can not suture a moving target very accurately, there is now more tendency to use general anaesthetics when suturing wounds. Having a steady operation site, without the need to beware of kicks etc. can give a better result and cut almost hours off the time taken to treat a wound.

Not every wound which is sutured will end up healing by first intention. It is, however, obviously better to suture a wound, say, 25 cm/10 in long and only have 10–15 cm/4–6 in

heal by first intention than it is to leave the whole length of the wound to heal by second intention. Not only that, but even where the sutures do not hold properly, they usually stabilize the skin and restrict the amount of gaping found in the wound. If a sutured wound does break down, any resulting granulation tissue must be contained level with the surrounding skin, because skin will not readily grow uphill. There are various chemical means of reducing proud flesh, but in some cases surgical removal may be advisable and quicker.

Stable hygiene and management

Make sure that your paddock is free of poisonous weeds and rubbish and that the fences are strong, preferably not of barbed wire. Keep your yard clear of objects which could cause accidents, and keep it well swept. Cleanliness is as important in the stable as it is in the home. Dirty wet straw decays in the stable and produces ideal conditions for bacteria to grow and multiply. At the ground level, neglecting to keep the stable bedding clean and dry can allow thrush to establish itself in the soft horn of the horse's frog.

When a horse recovers from an infection, the stable should be completely cleaned out and disinfected. It doesn't matter that you cannot see any infected remains, such as dried excreta etc., disinfection is still necessary. Drying is also a very effective method of killing bacteria and viruses.

There are some circumstances where general horsemastership can affect the spread of disease. Wherever possible, for instance, each horse should have his own grooming kit. This limits the spread of skin infections such as ringworm. From time to time the grooming kit should be cleaned in a solution of hot bleach. Whilst on the topic of spreading infection, mention should be made of isolation. I'm afraid that in most cases there is little point in removing infected horses to isolation quarters. By the time you realize the horse is ill, any spread of infection will already have occurred. It is, however, important not to allow fresh horses into the stable yard, or move horses out of the yard because that would expose them to additional risks of infection.

Drugs, their use and abuse

In preparing for later chapters which deal with specific ailments and their treatment I thought it would be useful to discuss some of the main classes of drugs which are used in veterinary medicine, and thus avoid some duplication. Three groups of drugs, namely the antibiotics, the corticosteroids and the non-steroidal anti-inflammatory agents, all have a variety of uses and so it is important to understand their exact effects in the horse's body.

ANTIBIOTICS

Antibiotics are substances which have an adverse effect on bacteria. They have no effect whatsoever on viruses. In some cases the antibiotic may actually kill the bacteria, and it is then said to be bactericidal. Penicillin is an example of a bactericidal antibiotic. Other antibiotics prevent any further reproduction of the bacteria, with the result that the numbers present decline due to 'old age'. These are said to be bacteriostatic antibiotics, of which the tetracyclines are perhaps the best known. Although you will not be involved in choosing which antibiotic to use in any given situation, some knowledge of these differences may be useful. Because bacteriostatic drugs do not actually kill the bacteria it is especially important that adequate drug levels are continually present if they are to be effective. As bacteria can double their numbers as frequently as every 30 or 40 minutes, even 2 or 3 hours without any drug present in the bloodstream can enable an infection to multiply. With bactericidal drugs the drug levels may not be so important, and dosing may not be quite so critical.

Because horses rely on friendly bacteria in the large bowel to carry out some digestion of the cellulose etc. in their diets which human beings, for example, cannot digest, antibiotics are not usually given to horses by mouth. Giving them in this way would obviously kill off the friendly bacteria resident in the bowels, as well as the unfriendly bacteria in some more remote part of the body which they were intended to kill. The majority of antibiotics are therefore given by injection. The length of time for which the antibiotic is active in the horse's body after an injection varies from drug to drug, and it is this which determines the frequency of dosage required. We are only just realizing that horses break down drugs at different rates to other animals of comparable size. A dose of long-acting penicillin will last four or five days in a cow, but the same dose would only be effective for two days in a horse. Similarly a single dose of a penicillin/streptomycin mixture will last 24 hours in a cow, but only perhaps for half that time in a horse. If we are to obtain the greatest benefit from these often expensive drugs, we must use them scientifically, not just economically.

CORTICOSTEROIDS

The corticosteroids (also referred to as the cortisones, or just as the steroids) reduce inflammation in the body. So where the classic signs of inflammation, namely pain, heat and swelling, are present, the corticosteroids may well be used. Valuable though this effect on inflammation is, we must remember that these symptoms are part of the body's defence mechanism, and we must be careful not to leave the body defenceless. The corticosteroids reduce all aspects of the body's defences, including those involved with fighting infections. This means that we would not normally use corticosteroids in a horse which we had just vaccinated, because the drug would reduce the beneficial development of immunity following vaccination. Nor would we use corticosteroids on their own in cases where infections were or could be present, as the infection would find it much easier to establish itself while the body's defences were muzzled. In this latter case it is customary to give antibiotics at the same time when corticosteroid treatment is essential. Corticosteroids are not pain killers. Because pain is often the result of inflammation, the use of these drugs will often appear, as an end result, to reduce pain but that is not a direct effect of the drugs themselves.

PHENYLBUTAZONE

In contrast, many of the anti-inflammatory drugs which are not steroids do have a direct analgesic or pain-relieving effect. Phenylbutazone (often referred to as 'bute') is perhaps the commonest, and also one of the cheapest, of these drugs available for use in horses. Flunixin meglumine, meclofenamic acid and naproxen are other examples of this type of drug. Generally speaking these drugs have a more powerful anti-inflammatory effect than the corticosteroids, especially in bone and muscle problems.

Anti-inflammatory drugs are not, however, without their side-effects. Although the non-steroidal anti-inflammatory drugs have less depressant effect on the horse's fight against infection than the corticosteroids, some effect still remains. Phenylbutazone, often used in the long-term relief of various arthritic conditions in the horse, has now been shown to be relatively toxic, especially in ponies. The moral is 'follow the instructions carefully'. Never be tempted to give higher doses than advised by your veterinary surgeon (veterinarian) because you will not obtain any better response, and never use these drugs without veterinary advice.

The availability of powerful drugs such as phenylbutazone has posed a problem for the authorities involved in regulating the various equine competitive fields. Their philosophy in this field might well be said to be that the use of drugs should not give one competitor an unfair advantage over another. The actual stance taken varies from country to country and from sport to sport. The British racing authority, the Jockey Club, bans the use of all drugs at any level. In America, on the other hand, some states ban all drugs but others allow the use of phenylbutazone as long as this is openly declared. At the present time Federal legislation is threatened to ban the use of all drugs from racing in America. The International Equestrian Federation (F.E.I.), which legislates for non-racing competitions such as horse trials, dressage and show-jumping, introduced new veterinary rules in 1981. Under these rules the use of any drug was prohibited, unless the drug was on a new list of 'permitted substances'. At present the only drug on this list is phenylbutazone, which must not be present at levels higher than four micrograms per millilitre of blood. But it is really necessary to establish levels for individual horses. No doubt the controversy will still continue as to whether any particular drug enables a horse to perform better than he should, or whether it merely enables the horse to regain its own previous pre-injury levels of performance.

4 A guide to feeding

The alimentary tract explained

The horse is a comparatively large animal, so the sheer bulk of bowels in the abdomen is considerable. The alimentary tract is a single tube which passes from the mouth through to the rectum. The design of this tube, unfortunately, often gives the impression that it has been designed by an amateur plumber, so prone is it to problems (as I will explain later). Once the horse has consciously swallowed a quantity of food, he has no further voluntary control over its passage along the tube until the faeces are ready to be passed out at the other end. Movement of food along the tract is by repeated rhythmic contractions which push the solids along.

The oesophagus (gullet) runs from the horse's mouth, down the neck and into the stomach. One point to notice is that although the walls of the oesophagus are capable of being stretched, there is a point where it passes into the thorax between two adjacent ribs. Obviously there is a limit to the size of solid mass which can pass along this section of the tube. The horse's stomach, which is comparatively small, lies at the front of the abdomen within the rib cage. One important detail is that the entrance to the stomach is very much a non-return valve, and the horse cannot vomit or regurgitate food except in very extreme circumstances. It is in the stomach that most digestion of carbohydrates occurs. Carbohydrates are the starchy foods which, when broken down during digestion, release energy. Most of this energy is used for maintaining the horse's normal activities. Any excess will be stored, either as fat, which may be formed throughout the horse's body for long term storage, or as glycogen. Glycogen is a readily accessible form of energy substance which is stored in the liver and in the muscles ready for immediate use.

After leaving the stomach food passes into the small intestine which, although lying predominantly in the anterior (front) part of the abdomen, is very much the 'filler' occupying space around larger organs. Most of the digestion of proteins occurs in the horse's small intestine. Proteins are, of course, vital because they are the building blocks for muscle etc. The small intestines end in the ileo-caecal valve at the entrance to the caecum. The horse's caecum is not a small insignificant organ like the appendix which is the human equivalent, but a large pear-shaped organ occupying most of the right flank.

The remainder of the alimentary tract, from the caecum to the rectum, is taken up by the large colon. In the colon are a large number of 'friendly bacteria' which have a life of their own and yet live permanently inside the horse. Actually there is a mixture of different types of bacteria, each living on a different type of food. So bacteria in the horse's colon break down food substances to produce extremely simple forms of carbohydrate, which the horse then absorbs through the walls of the colon for his own use. Some proteins are obtained in a similar way, but the main function of these bacteria is to break

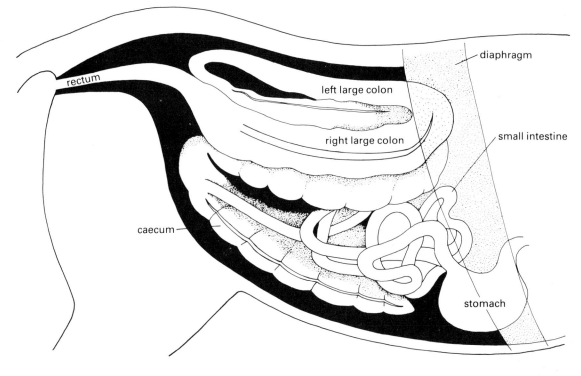

The digestive tract.

down the cellulose found in all plant material with which ordinary mammalian digestions such as those found in the cat or dog, cannot cope. In order to provide sufficient volume for all this bacterial activity the colon needs to be a large organ. It starts at the caecum in the right flank and passes forward to the diaphragm, where it does a U-turn so that it is running backwards along the left flank. Right at the rear of the abdomen is the so-called 'pelvic flexure', where the colon turns sharply through 180° before paralleling its path (this time lying on top of its original portion) back to the right flank and then the rectum. So the large colon of the horse is rather like two hoops lying one on top of another and joined together at their left-hand ends. As if this was not complicated enough, the upper hoop has a much smaller diameter than the lower one, and this change of diameter occurs just as the colon is turning back on itself at the pelvic flexure. No wonder the horse suffers from bowel problems!

What to feed and why

If one were to ask the average British town dweller what was a horse's staple food, he would probably answer 'Oats and grass'. In fact oats are only one of many cereals which can be fed to horses. They actually have a lower starch and energy content than either barley, wheat, maize (corn in the USA), or sorghum (USA). Oats do not require any processing before feeding to horses, whereas cereals such as barley or wheat should be rolled before feeding. This process breaks open the kernel of the cereal. One reason for the popularity of oats as a food for horses over the centuries has been the fact that their weight and their energy content per unit volume is relatively low and so there is less danger of overfeeding problems than if wheat, for example is used. In addition, wheat contains gluten, making it a pasty mass in the intestine.

In addition to energy, cereals can also supply the basic 'maintenance' requirements for crude proteins in adult horses. More usually, however, a horse which is not in active work would receive over half (in weight) of its diet as hay or grass. The contents of hay obviously vary enormously. They vary from haystack to haystack in one village, from farm to farm in an area and they vary from country to country, and from state to state, because the proportions of the various grasses and herbs (legumes in USA) present varies with what grows well in the prevailing climate. In Britain hay usually has about 4% to 7% crude protein. In the USA it has 8% to 16%. It is worth observing that where the protein content is low, protein digestibility also tends to be low, so feeding poor quality hay results in even less protein being actually available to the horse than you would perhaps expect.

As we will see later the presence or absence of fibre can cause problems for the horse's alimentary tract. As in all young animals, young growing horses need large quantities of the 'building block' proteins. Youngsters should thus be given the most digestible foods, and dietary protein supplements may sometimes be advisable.

Minerals

Much has been said and written about the mineral requirements of horses, especially the calcium and phosphorus requirements. Adequate calcium is essential if bone of the correct strength and density is to be formed. Paradoxically, feeding too much phosphorus will markedly decrease the amount of calcium absorbed from the intestines (no matter what quantities of calcium may have been originally present in the food), but feeding excess calcium has relatively little effect on absorbtion of phosphorus *(see page 30)*. It has now been shown that whenever there is a choice, horses will tend to graze the hard grasses (which have low calcium levels) rather than the good quality grass/legume mixtures (which contain more calcium). It only goes to show that horses have little nutritional wisdom.

Vitamins

Horse owners also worry about the vitamins which their horses are receiving. As cereals and good quality grazing/hay contain adequate levels of the vitamin B group, and as the bacteria in the colon synthesise these vitamins as well, it is unlikely that any deficiencies will occur. Folic acid can, however, be lacking in stabled horses and in mares after foaling. Access to really good grazing, especially that with a good legume content, will solve any such problems. Horse diets are, however, occasionally low in vitamin A, and vitamin D levels may also be low, especially where little hay is fed and when the horse is not exposed to the bright sunlight necessary for it to manufacture vitamin D in its skin.

Hay and grazing obviously constitute quite a large proportion of a horse's diet, and certainly provide a significant proportion of his energy requirements. Hay can vary enormously in quality. Good legume hay such as lucerne (alfalfa in USA) hay provides more energy than a corresponding grass hay. On the other hand poorer quality lucerne (alfalfa) hay will contain more mould and dust, and less leaf, than grass hay. Lucerne (alfalfa) hay is rich in protein, and so an abrupt change to lucerne (alfalfa) hay can cause a digestive upset. Changeovers from one type of hay to another, or from one year's hay to another, should always be carried out gradually. Because lucerne (alfalfa) hay is a good, though in Britain often expensive, source of calcium, horses receiving significant quantities of it may well pass a rather cloudy urine. This cloudiness is due to certain calcium salts and is not a cause for concern.

The inter-relationship between protein and fibre digestibility is important. This certainly applies to grazing. Following rain in the late spring and early autumn, pastures have a high leaf content and a higher protein content. During the dry summer period the less digestible flower stems make up more of the pasture, and horses with a high protein requirement, e.g. mares feeding a foal, will require some extra protein. Horses should always have access to either grazing or hay for some part of the day.

One factor which many horse owners fail to realize is that it is not necessarily a good thing for a horse to finish its feed too quickly. A slower rate of eating may improve digestibility and reduce boredom, as long as chewing is not merely being slowed down by tooth problems. Chopped hay (or straw) takes longer to eat than long hay, and the use of such 'chaff' is regaining popularity in Britain. Similarly, ground cereals, although more dusty, take longer to eat than crushed cereals and pellets.

Certain foods, such as bran and sugar beet pulp, absorb large quantities of water, and so prevent 'bolting' of food when they are fed wet. Their very bulk prevents overloading of the digestive tract with large quantities of dry matter. I emphasize the need to soak sugar beet pulp or nuts overnight, as otherwise dry portions of the pulp can swell rapidly due to absorbtion of saliva while passing down the oesophagus and may cause an oesophageal obstruction. Feeding unsoaked sugar beet is the main cause of choking in horses and ponies. I should mention here that horses can only produce saliva whilst actually chewing. It follows, therefore, that a food which requires little chewing, e.g. cereals, will contain less fluid. It will also contain less salivary salts, and without these salts the bowel contents tend to become more and more acid until the balance of bacteria in the colon becomes upset. Water should, of course, always be available for all horses. Not only is it necessary to replace fluid lost as saliva, urine, sweat etc., but also for absorbtion with the bowel contents, as we have seen.

I will not try to lay down firm rules as to what you should feed your horse. This will depend so much on where you live, what is available, what work your horse is required to perform, and the size of your horse or pony. Nor is it possible to deal with all the various supplementary feeds which may be added to a horse's staple diet. Milk powder, for instance, has become increasingly popular, although not always for the correct reasons. People naturally assume that milk powder or milk pellets have a good calcium and phosphorus content for building strong bones. What is not realized is that they contain only slightly more calcium than hay, and less than some other foods e.g. sugar beet pulp. So balancing a horse's diet can be a very complicated process. Unless you have a reasonable amount of experience, I would urge you to stick to a basic hay/proprietary horse cubes diet and follow the manufacturer's instructions. Reputable manufacturers can utilize a range of ingredients which the average horse owner of only one or two horses could not possibly justify. Or, in the USA, feed a hay/grain and/or pellets diet, with grain and pellets never more than half the total weight eaten.

The following contains some additional guidelines and suggestions.

A background to feeding in Britain

In Britain, feeding of the stabled horse is traditionally based on grass hay, oats (usually crushed) and bran. To many horse owners these are the only feeds they will ever consider using. Others use some barley (rolled or cooked), maize (corn in USA) (flaked, and more recently micronized), feed beans and peas, linseed (tea and jelly) and soaked sugar beet pulp. Other feedstuffs enjoying varying degrees of popularity include grass meal or nuts (a much neglected, versatile food which I hope will increase in usage), lucerne (alfalfa in USA) meal and nuts, soya bean meal and skimmed milk powder.

Sugar beet pulp or nuts, which must be soaked for 12 hours before feeding, tends to be more readily available in the eastern part of Britain, near the beet factories, and in the past this has also applied to dried grass although currently the south and south-west is better supplied in this commodity. Being in different protein/energy grades, it can be used as part of the concentrate ration, or part of the forage portion of the diet, where the cubes are especially suited to the horse with respiratory problems.

CEREALS
MAIZE AND BARLEY
In Britain, maize (corn in USA) is virtually never fed whole or on the cob, but always steam-flaked, or more recently micronized, a process which appears to make it (and any other cereals or legumes thus treated) more digestible and therefore increase its food value. Barley is, and should be, fed rolled or cooked, and is regaining popularity. It is a feed which suffers from a number of misconceptions – but provided it is fed as part of a *balanced* diet there is no reason why barley should not form the sole cereal

constituent of the diet. Unfortunately many people try to use maize and barley substituted for oats directly on a weight for weight basis. They are not the same and this a sure recipe for unbalancing the diet. Oats contain more fibre (and calcium) than maize or barley, but less energy (which is why 'weight for weight' they are less fattening). Oats are particularly deficient in an important 'amino acid', lysine, although none of the cereals contain very high levels.

OATS

Very few people in Britain feed whole oats, although there is little nutritional advantage in rolling, bruising or crushing them for a mature horse or pony. Unless you are rolling daily, any slight advantage in digestibility is cancelled out by loss in feeding value due to oxidation of vitamins, and even growth of moulds, and the cost in time, money and machinery of rolling them. It is worth remembering that a whole oat is alive, and would grow if you planted it, a rolled one is dead, and dead things decay rapidly. If you buy-in oats ready-rolled, do not buy more than you can use in 14 days, and ensure they are fresh-rolled. The only animals worth the trouble and expense of rolled oats are those under 6 months of age, and elderly horses with worn teeth. 'Clipped oats' have had part of the fibrous seed coat knocked off, so have a higher nutritional value than unclipped oats, but this needs to be justified from the cost point of view.

CHAFF, OR CHOP

Chaff or chop, i.e. chopped hay or straw, especially oat straw, was very popular in years gone by, and after virtually disappearing for 20 years or so, has regained popularity in the last 2–3 years, with the introduction in Britain of four or five new chaff-cutting machines of various sizes – not a moment too soon as old-style chaff cutters had become 'worth their weight in gold' if you could find one. Chaff is a useful way of slowing down eating, encouraging the horse to chew its food properly and of getting some forage into a high performance horse with a limited appetite for hay alone.

BRAN

Wheat bran, especially 'broad bran' has been gradually disappearing from the food market, as wheat milling has become more efficient (it is, after all, a by-product), and is much lamented by many traditionalists in the horsey community. They say it isn't what it was in grandfather's day, which is true; but conveniently forget that it was not even used until the 1850s or later, when white bread first became available on a wide scale! However, I see no real reason to mourn the passing of bran. For bulk and fibre in the ration we have grass meal (*much* better from a nutritional point of view), or chaff. If we feed a balanced diet we should not need to feed bran mashes. Bran has a most unfavourable calcium: phosphorus ratio (low in calcium and high in phosphorus); and also contains a substance called phytate (phytin, phytic acid) which 'locks up' calcium in the diet and prevents the horse from absorbing it in the gut. If a lot of bran is fed this can lead to serious bone abnormalities, including 'big-head' or 'bran-disease' which manifests itself as bony enlargements of the head, which has a puffy swollen appearance. So no horse should ever be fed a lot of bran.

Additional protein

Cereals really supply all the protein a mature riding horse needs, but more protein, of a higher quality, is required for the young growing animal, the pregnant mare in the last 90 days of gestation, and in lactation, and to a degree for the very high performance horse, which I believe benefits from improved protein quality, to ensure potentially deficient amino acids such as lysine and methionine are provided.

The additional protein may be supplied using skimmed milk, white fish meal, meat and bone meal, soya bean meal, cottonseed meal, linseed, feed beans and peas. I prefer not to use animal proteins apart from milk powder. Of the plant proteins soya bean meal has the best amino acid makeup, then cottonseed (more widely used in the USA than Britain). Linseed has a rather unbalanced amino acid makeup. It can be fed as oilcake, or the seed can (and *must* be) cooked to give a 'jelly and tea'. Given the dubious protein quality I consider the latter process a waste of time unless an animal is suffering from a digestive disorder which requires the lubricating qualities of the jelly in the digestive tract. Stockfeed beans and peas were popular winter feed for cart horses in days gone by, and current EEC policy towards their production should see them being used more widely in Britain. They contain about half the protein of soya bean, but are a valuable energy source.

FORAGE
HAY

On the forage side, I think the next decade will see marked changes in horse feeding in Britain. Grass hay is the main forage source, but as fewer and fewer livestock farmers produce grass hay, as dairy and beef farmers change over to silage (basically 'pickled grass'), the average horse owner finds that not only does his local farm source no longer grow hay, they no longer keep the machinery to 'pop along' and cut the horse owner's few acres either. As this movement grows in an area, the local agricultural contractors no longer keep haymaking equipment, not worth their while for a few acres of horse paddocks. So the owner of just a few acres can no longer grow his own hay economically, and finds it increasingly difficult to buy it locally.

The hay which is available is generally barn-dried, which usually means it is a better quality than most field-cured (i.e. dried) hay which has either been sun-scorched, or rain-soaked (which washes the soluble nutrients out and encourages moulds) or both. The virtues of sun-cured hay are often exaggerated and only the best samples are worth all the fuss; especially if you then store the hay for a year or even two before use, by which time almost all the vitamins will have disappeared and a good deal of the protein. Most people, even 'good hay judges' are sadly disappointed when they see an analysis of their hay.

The main thing to look for in hay is that it is leafy (therefore higher in protein) and devoid of dust and mould and poisonous weeds. This applies to both grass and legume hays. If possible buy from a farmer or merchant who has his hay analysed – the price will probably still be based on local market conditions rather than actual hay quality, but at least you will *know* what you are feeding and be able to balance it with confidence instead of guesswork. If you grow your own hay, or buy in large quantities it is worth having an analysis done yourself.

Lucerne (alfalfa in USA) hay is not widely available in Britain as we do not have the best weather conditions for its cultivation. What is available is often of poor quality due to bad (wet) weather at harvest. However, it is available in some areas, as is sainfoin hay, another legume. I think in the future we shall see another legume hay, called fenugreek, become popular for horses in this country. All the legume hays have a generally higher protein content than grass hays, and more calcium (hence the cloudy urine often seen when it is fed in large quantities).

Other hays in Britain are seed hay (ryegrass and red clover) and meadow hay (mixed grasses and clovers including wild white clover, and possibly some herbs). The problem with mixed grass and legume hays is that they are more inclined to mould as the two types of plants cure at different rates. I prefer to use separately grown grass and legumes and mix them at feeding-time.

In the absence of hay – either due to price, unavailability, or allergy (the horse and/or handler may be allergic to hay), five years ago the prospects seemed bleak. Now, a number of alternatives are presenting themselves as practical propositions. These are silage, 'Haylage', dried grass and lucerne as nuts and meal, and oat and barley straw and ground ammonia or alkali-treated straw.

SILAGE, PARTICULARLY GRASS SILAGE

Grass for silage is cut at an earlier and more nutritious stage than grass for hay. However, it is wetter and bulkier than hay so is not really suitable as a significant forage source for high performance horses – except as a refreshing succulent. It also 'spoils' rapidly on exposure to air, so needs to be cut and stored near to where it will be fed. Once they are accustomed to the taste, horses seem to prefer silage to hay. Silage is less dependent on the weather when it is being made than hay, but it may be 'wilted' before storage, which makes it less bulky, and wilted silage is to be preferred for horse feeding. To date, most silage fed to horses has been mixed 50:50 with hay or straw, or if it is self-fed from a silage clamp, hay or straw is also offered.

Silage needs to be eaten near where it is stored, so, unless you have a farm, may not be practical. However, in Britain, farmers are now making silage, especially on sheep farms, in large round bales, which are stored and sealed in large plastic bags. It would be possible to ship these locally, so that a horse owner with limited storage space could buy a few 'bales' at a time.

Maize (corn in the USA) silage is also being fed to horses in Europe but little specific information is as yet available about this.

'HAYLAGE' or 'HAYAGE'

Another alternative is forage ensiled in a tower silo. There is some confusion over what this should be called as the most popular name for this material, 'Haylage' is copyright of the makers of one particular type of silo. However, the product is between hay and silage in quality and dry matter.

Another grass product has the confusingly similar name of 'Horseage'. In this case the grass is just cut at a predetermined moisture and protein content and vacuum-pressure packed in a sealed polythene bag, i.e. there is no wilting or ensiling. There is some variation in the quality of different brands, but in principle they are a good idea, and usually justify their cost far better than importing hay in bad hay years. They were introduced for animals with hay allergies, but are favoured by increasing numbers of performance horse trainers who wish to minimize even possible non-clinical stress to their valuable horses' (and handlers') respiratory systems.

The grass is cut at the optimum time so these products tend to be higher in protein and digestible energy content than most hay. This means in many cases, for a least the average riding horse, the concentrate ration may be correspondingly reduced. They also come with a guaranteed analysis on the bag, so you can formulate a properly balanced ration – instead of guessing the food value. Care should be taken not to puncture the bags, which should be used within three to four days of opening.

DRIED GRASS AND LUCERNE

Other major hay alternatives, already mentioned, are dried grass and dried lucerne, both of which are available as meal or nuts. They are a very logical food for horses and are particularly useful for animals with respiratory problems. There is sometimes an initial problem with palatability, but gradual introduction, and the judicious use (as a last resort) of apple juice, molasses or molassine meal should overcome

this, and once converted, most horses are loth to go back to hay. Careful handling is advisable as these products easily break into 'dust'.

OAT AND BARLEY STRAW

Good quality oat or barley straw may also be fed. I like to soak barley straw to soften any prickly awns which may be present. Straw is especially useful feed as chaff or chop. There is a lot of straw wasted in Britain and much of it is of better quality than so-called 'horse hay'. Straw may also be processed, i.e. ground and treated with alkali or ammonia – I have no information about feeding the tubground product to horses, but one major food compounder produces a branded cubed alkali-treated straw, which again is sold by analysis, and has performed trials in feeding horses. I think this product holds great promise, and the alkali *could* have specifically beneficial effects on high performance horses on high energy diets, prone to varying degrees of acidosis, especially if an unexpected lay-off occurs.

PRESERVATIVES

Whether dealing with hay or silage, or even grain, especially in bad weather years, preservatives are increasingly used. There are various types, but little information on their effect on horses. The exception is proprionic acid (e.g. 'Propcorn') which is quite safe for horses, but increases the need for vitamin E in the diet, so a high-vitamin E (alpha-tocopherol) supplement should be fed in this situation.

Supplements

In Britain, the main basic supplements required are salt (in most cases a trace-mineralized salt-lick is adequate, but the high performance horse should have salt added to the concentrate ration), calcium (when grass hays are fed) e.g. as limestone (calcium carbonate) and vitamins A and D. The stabled horse which has no access to pasture at all is also likely to benefit from B-vitamins, including folacin (folate, folic acid) and biotin (also called vitamin H), and vitamins C, E and K, plus trace minerals which should include selenium and zinc (Se and Zn), and if necessary amino acids lysine and methionine. The pregnant mare, lactating mare, and young-stock all have different requirements, in both amount and proportion of nutrients, and for example it is now becoming clear that vitamin C is more important in the diet of youngstock under the age of 6 months than was previously realized.

When thinking of nutrition, it is worth remembering that young racehorses may still be growing as well as working, and likewise brood mares may still be growing. Elderly horses should also not be forgotten. They may have difficulty chewing, and require rolled or cooked cereals and succulent pasture. They may also have different vitamin and mineral requirements to younger animals.

A background to feeding in the USA

In the USA, of course the principles of feeding are the same as in Britain, but variations in environment, including extremes of heat and cold, and available feedstuffs, mean there are fundamental differences in some instances.

CEREALS

Sorghum (milo) and millet are two cereals not even heard of by many British horse owners, which enjoy some popularity as grains, and in the case of sorghum, forage as well, for horses in the USA. Corn (maize in Britain) is very widely fed, frequently either on the cob in growing regions, or removed from the cob, as whole grain. Alfalfa (lucerne) hay is also more widely used, and as it has a high calcium and protein content, and corn (maize) is low in both these nutrients, a corn and alfalfa (lucerne) hay diet is a popular combination.

Oats, usually fed whole, barley and grass hay, and grass/clover mixtures are of course also fed, and vary in type and nutritional value depending on the climate, soil type and grass variety used in different regions.

Regional variations in grain usage usually depend on local growing conditions, or proximity to ports (such as Bristol, Erith, Hull and Liverpool in Britain). Current varieties of oats grow best in cool, moist climates such as north-western America, Scotland and the north of England. Barley is widely grown in all except the hottest, most humid regions. Food value of maize (corn) is subject to wide regional variations, but the crop seems to prefer sandy, well-drained soil.

Regional and climatic variations

Discussion of regional grass and hay varieties is beyond the scope of this book, but look for plenty of leaf, cut or grazed at the optimum time, and the absence of poisonous weeds.

Extremes of temperatures influence nutrition in a number of ways. Extreme cold obviously increases the energy requirement for maintenance of body condition. It may also mean an animal is kept indoors, or at least covered by rugs and exercise rugs, for many months of the year, which means reduced exposure to sunlight which is needed for conversion of vitamin D in the skin. Dietary vitamin D should be increased.

There are riding schools and livery yards in some areas, where the horses are stabled in barns attached to indoor arenas, and may barely set foot out of doors for 4–6 months of the year. This type of animal is likely to be especially prone to respiratory disorders, especially if ventilation is poor, and artificial heat is used – often to prevent water from freezing – and for the benefit of humans! Feeding and bedding may therefore be adjusted to reduce airborne dust and moulds in this type of environment.

At another extreme, in hot, dry (arid) regions, including for example the mid-western prairies, many plants are unable to take up minerals effectively from the soil, so grazed grass, and even hay and grain from these regions, may be deficient in certain nutrients. Hay grown in drought conditions generally tends to be low in phosphorus in particular, and further than this, excess calcium occurs in the soil of the arid western regions, so phosphorus must be added to the diet, or offered to grazing animals with a suitable, local mineral mixture and salt.

Salt requirements may be higher in hot, dry conditions, certainly for animals which sweat for any reason, and apart from common salt (sodium chloride), magnesium and potassium salts may also be required for the performance animal. These 'blood salts' are also called electrolytes, and electrolyte supplementation of endurance horses competing for example for the Tevis Cup, is becoming a specialized subject in its own right. Vitamin C requirements also appear to increase in very hot conditions, and I suspect there are other variations in vitamin and mineral requirements which will come to light.

Regional deficiencies and excesses of nutrients

In Britain, from the horse's point of view, there are not yet vast tracts of land exceptionally deficient, or even over-supplied, with specific nutrients, although I believe there are more inter-relationships between certain disease conditions and soil types than we are as yet fully aware of. However, in the USA, over 40 states have been identified as having soil markedly deficient in selenium, a tendency with acid soils, although there are areas of the Rocky Mountains and 'Great Plains States', with alkaline soil conditions, where highly toxic levels of selenium are present.

Another trace element which may suffer regional variations is iodine, which may be present in excess on pastures and hays in coastal and small island areas, where iodized salt, and seaweed supplements may have to be avoided, but may be severely deficient in so called 'goitre belts', such as Derbyshire in north-east England, and California, Colorado, Dakota (N. and S.), Illinois, Indiana, Iowa, Michigan, Montana, Nebraska, Nevada, New York, Ohio, Oregon, Utah, Washington and Wisconsin. In these areas iodized salt should be fed. Both deficiency and excess of iodine can lead to goitre (an enlarged thyroid gland), even in newborn foals whose mother's diets are unbalanced.

With this, and other possible mineral imbalances in mind, I would suggest it is worthwhile using regional formulations of compound feeds or vitamin and mineral supplements, for your particular region, rather than choosing a 'national' brand which is not varied in composition for different areas. Check this out with your feed dealer.

Wherever you are it makes sound sense to take the time and trouble to find out what is in your foodstuffs, even if you can only find out where they were grown and any prevalent deficiencies or excesses in the region, and to balance those foodstuffs for your horse and the work it is expected to perform.

COTTONSEED CAKE AND MOLASSES

Cottonseed cake is more freely available as a protein source in the US than Britain; and another feedstuff widely used to keep down dust and improve palatability is molasses. In the US this is more likely to mean cane (sugar cane) molasses whereas in Britain it means beet (sugar beet) molasses.

MANIOC

A cereal substitute appearing in both countries, mainly in compound foods, is manioc (or tapioca, or cassava), a root product which is safe for horse feeding. However, it is sometimes supplied in a pelleted form, when cocoa bean meal *may* be used to raise the protein level. This product should not be used for horses, as cocoa bean from any source (including cake/biscuit/confectionery waste) contains caffeine and theobromine, which are non-permitted substances for horses competing under Jockey Club and FEI rules, as well as many national and state horse sport and showing organizations.

GRASS MATS

A 'forage alternative' not yet seen in Britain, but available in the USA, which we shall probably see more of, is a 'grass' (more often oats/rye/barley) grown hydroponically (in water) in trays in environmentally controlled 'huts'. These form a grass 'mat', which is fed roots and all, as a fresh forage source, each mat taking around 7 days to go from sowing to feeding stage. This has the advantage of producing a highly nutritious succulent, dust and disease free food in a small area all the year round and will be especially attractive to horse owners in urban areas, and for horses with respiratory problems.

Commercial horse feeds

(Compound horse feeds in Britain, formula feeds in USA)

These terms cover a number of types of food formulated by a feed mill to provide a balanced diet for a specific group of horses. In general they should take into account regional variations in forage and other foodstuffs, and will be covered by a label declaration of at least part of their food value. Compound feeds may be pelleted (pellets, nuts or cubes) or coarse mixes.

Pellets may be 'complete' – i.e. contain both the forage and grain part of the ration. These are useful for horses with respiratory problems, but are inflexible unless you have a customized mix; and what is suitable for the pleasure horse may be inadequate for a racehorse or showjumper.

Work load of horse	Weight of feed Forage	Grain/cubes	Pellet type
Light work	60–75%	25–30%	Horse & Pony
Medium work	50%	50%	Manufacturers' instructions
Brood mare	50%	50%	Stud
Hard work	25–30%	60–75%	Racehorse
	100%		'Complete cubes'

They can also lead to vices due to boredom in a few animals, but are reportedly widely used in south-western USA (e.g. Arizona) where pasture is poor and scarce due to low rainfall.

Other pellets are forage balancers, of different formulations – e.g. 'Horse & Pony', 'Hunter', 'Stud', 'Racehorse' cubes etc. It is important to remember that these are only balanced when used as the manufacturer intended. If you 'dilute' them with other foods, you unbalance them. If you use a 'Racehorse' cube instead of 'Horse and Pony', not only will you feed the wrong type, but the manufacturer will assume you base your feeding as in the table above:

This table is a general 'rule of thumb' and a food manufacturer will use it just as you should.

The third type of pellet is a 'protein concentrate' or 'grain balancer'. Here the manufacturer assumes you feed forage and some grain, and provides you with a high-protein cube (usually 25% crude protein for horses) with vitamins and minerals added to balance the *whole feed*.

Coarse rations

These are generally forage balancers, and are unpelleted compound foods. They are becoming quite popular in Britain, where horse owners wish to use a mixed food they know is balanced, but like to 'see what is in it'. The term is used in Britain to cover grain mixtures, ranging to sophisticated cereal and legume mixes, with pelleted vitamins minerals and proteins added. In the USA, the terminology is more precise, and could be usefully adopted in Britain.

US coarse mixes are either sweetfeed or textured feeds.

SWEETFEED

This consists of highly molassed cereals including perhaps rolled barley, corn (flaked, rolled or whole) and oats. Protein may also be added as soya bean meal, cottonseed cake or linseed cake, plus a vitamin and mineral pellet. In Britain I have also seen locust bean meal, split peas and beans used, and the barley, maize, peas and beans may be micronized. The oats are generally crushed in British mixes.

TEXTURIZED FEEDS

These are similar to sweetfeed, but with up to 60% pellets which contain protein as well as vitamins and minerals.

Changing your horse's feed

If you change your feeding, do so gradually, whether you are introducing a new ingredient – even only a spoonful of supplement, do so over 3–14 days – depending on what it is. This includes changing batches of hay, cereals, or brands of compound feeds. The micro-organisms in your horse's intestines need time to adjust to new food (including grazing) and chopping and changing can lead to colic, or metabolic disorders such as acidosis and laminitis. This applies to decreases as well as increases in food ingredients.

Water supply

Wherever and whatever you are feeding, you must ensure a constant supply of *fresh* water from a suitable outlet. This may be a natural spring or stream, but be sure there is no pollution entering upstream, that access is good, and that the bottom is firm, not sandy, as ingestion of sand can cause sand colic (*See page 38*). A stagnant pond is not suitable. Automatic-filling waterers should be checked daily to see they are working – and a meter is useful in a stable so you can tell how much the animal is drinking. (Non-drinking, or excessive water consumption are both signs that all is not well.) Clean out water troughs and buckets frequently. Do not just top-up stable buckets, empty and refill them at least twice a day. Standing water absorbs ammonia from the air (from urine in the stable) and becomes unpalatable. Some horses may become extremely thirsty before they will attempt to drink such water.

Problems associated with feeding

CHOKING (CHOKE IN USA)

As I have already mentioned, a horse only produces saliva during chewing. When it does so, however, quite large quantities of saliva are mixed with the food and swallowed. If certain foods, such as sugar beet pulp, are fed dry then they swell up rapidly during their passage down the oesophagus, or gullet, due to absorbtion of water from the saliva. The amount of swelling can be so great that the 'bolus' of food which was swallowed cannot pass any further down the oesophagus. The horse then has an oesophageal obstruction, or is said to be 'choked'. There are other ways in which such an obstruction can occur as well as by the rapid swelling of dry feed. If a horse bolts down large lumps of unchewed food such as carrots, then he may become choked. A horse can even become choked on quite normal food if some sudden surprise causes a reflex constriction and clamping down of the muscles along the oesophagus. In this case, by the time the horse has thought about relaxing, and letting the food pass on its way, a sufficient 'traffic jam' of food has accumulated to form a real obstruction.

A choked horse will obviously not be able to eat or drink, so you will see the horse standing looking miserable, with uneaten food in his manger. The gullet, or oesophagus gradually fills up with saliva, until the horse starts to drool saliva from his nose and mouth. One of the potential side effects with a choking horse is that some of this saliva may run down into the horse's lung, and start a pneumonia. Often you will be able to feel the blockage in the oesophagus as it runs down the furrow along the lower part of the horse's neck on the left hand side.

Although oesophageal obstructions will occasionally clear themselves, if it is of sufficient duration for saliva to be drooling from the horse's mouth then do not delay in obtaining veterinary assistance. Keep food and water away from the horse until the veterinary surgeon (veterinarian) arrives. Sometimes an injection of some form of muscle relaxant will be sufficient to allow the blockage to pass on its way down to the stomach. In other cases the veterinary surgeon (veterinarian) will use a stomach tube to free the obstruction. This is not done by just attempting to force the obstruction onwards, as this may well result in tearing the wall of the oesophagus. Instead the mass is alternately soaked with water and then this water, and hopefully some of the softened food mass, is pumped away with a stomach pump. The process is repeated until all the obstruction has been removed, which can take quite a time. Once the obstruction has been freed, the horse is completely recovered. The proof of this is that the horse can swallow water readily. Because some damage or scarring of the internal wall of the oesophagus can occur at the site of the obstruction, care is obviously needed in feeding over the next few days.

COLIC

Colic is, by definition, nothing more or less than abdominal pain. This abdominal pain is, however, a warning signal which brings the physician to the patient (whether animal or human), and it is nature's way of indicating that something is wrong. It is important that you recognize the varied ways in which the horse will react to colic and show his discomfort. The horse may paw the ground with his front legs, or kick his abdomen with his hind legs. If you feel the horse's abdomen it will feel hard and tense, and the horse will often sweat, either all over his body or just in odd patches. If the pain becomes more extreme the horse may become so anguished that he throws himself down on the ground and rolls violently in an attempt to relieve the pain. On the other hand, when the pain is less severe there may be very little in the way of symptoms. The horse may just be very dull and quite miserable, and be unwilling to eat its food.

Most of this abdominal pain is caused by distension or 'ballooning' of the bowels. Even where the underlying cause is a spasm, there is always a certain amount of dilation in the adjacent portions of the bowel. Normal bowel movements progress along in a rhythmic wave of contraction followed by relaxation. When the rhythm is upset, the waves may 'collide' with each other, causing peaks of pain. In cases of impaction, where bowel movement stops completely, there is a corresponding absence of any acute pain.

Impaction of the stomach

Impaction of the stomach usually occurs due to over-eating. As a result of bad management or accident the horse gains access to an appetizing food and eats until the stomach is so full and stretched that no muscular contractions can occur. It may also arise when large amounts of dry food swell up in the stomach due to absorbtion of saliva and stomach juices. If this happened in a human being, vomiting would occur in order to empty the stomach, but because the valve at the entrance to the horse's stomach is too small to allow any regurgitation, the horse cannot vomit.

Horses with an impaction of the stomach are in great pain. They will often sit back on their haunches, rather like the position of a dog sitting down, in an attempt to relieve the pressure of the other abdominal contents on the swollen stomach. Urgent treatment is essential. Do not delay, because all too often the end result with a stomach impaction is rupture of the stomach and death. Passage of a stomach tube may allow your veterinary surgeon (veterinarian) to relieve the pressure in the stomach in a similar way to that described with choking. If this fails, then surgery is the only hope.

A horse rolling in acute colic.

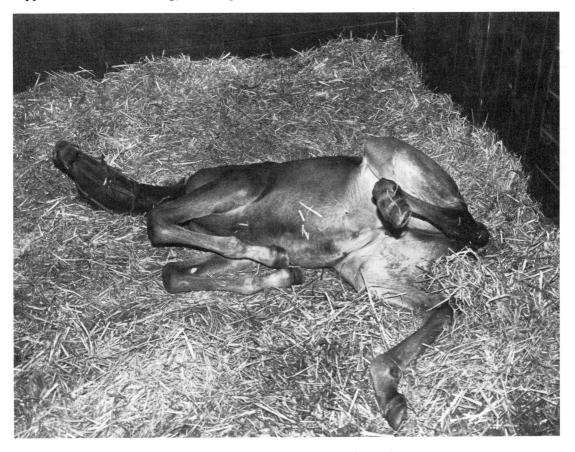

Intestinal impactions

Impaction of the small intestine gives rise to a chronic pain. The horse is dull, and may spend a lot of time lying absolutely flat out (almost as if it were dead) in the stable. Often the mucous membranes around the eyes are yellow due to jaundice. The hold up occurs most frequently at the valve where the small intestine joins the caecum.

Impactions of the large colon have very similar symptoms, although jaundice is not usually present in this case. The impaction almost always occurs at the pelvic flexure where, as I have explained, the colon not only bends through 180° but also drastically reduces its diameter. Veterinary surgeons (veterinarians) can often locate these impactions by inserting an arm into the horse's rectum and palpating the various internal organs.

Contrary to what you might at first think, horses with an intestinal impaction do not necessarily stop passing any faeces. This is because only rarely is movement stopped along the whole length of the alimentary tract, and any contents further behind than the actual impaction can still be passed. So if a horse with an impaction stops passing faeces, the condition has already existed for some little time. Such horses may strain frequently, but produce only small amounts of foul brown liquid.

Impactions arise due to the accumulation of coarse undigested food material. Feeding poor quality roughage is only asking for trouble, as it will not be chewed or digested properly. If a horse has dental problems, the roughage will not be properly chewed. Often the horse is simply incapable of properly digesting perfectly nutritious food. This happens if the horse has been accustomed to the high carbohydrate content of grass, and when a more fibrous material such as hay or straw is eaten instead, the horse lacks the right blend of bacteria inside his large colon to digest this food. The fibrous material accumulates within the large colon, and dries out as its moisture is absorbed, until it becomes impacted at the pelvic flexure and will pass no further. In the USA, ravelled rubber belting used for fencing has been eaten by some young horses, causing a particularly dangerous recurrent impaction.

Treatment of impactions is not a matter for the horse owner. Patent colic drinks or medicines are not only of no therapeutic value, the giving of liquids to a horse by mouth is dangerous. The chance of the horse getting some of the liquid down his trachea (wind-pipe) into his lungs is too great. Veterinary treatment has the dual aims of both softening the impacted mass, which otherwise becomes harder and harder as the body continues to absorb more moisture from it through the bowel wall, and secondly stimulating normal bowel movements in order to move the mass onwards towards the rectum.

The drugs used are called purgatives or purges, and there are two main types. Saline purgatives attract fluids from the bloodstream into the bowel in order to dilute the strong concentration of salt they contain. The increased bowel volume, coupled with the medication's softening effect, stimulates bowel movement. Because saline purgatives do increase the volume of bowel contents, they may not be suitable for repeated administration, which is only safely carried out via a stomach tube.

Oil-based purgatives such as mineral oil or liquid paraffin, on the other hand, act by causing a mild irritation of the bowel wall until bowel movements start again. Movement of the impacted mass along the rest of the length of bowels will always be slow. It can take several days of repeated treatments via stomach tube before success is achieved, and the horse owner must then have patience and confidence in his veterinary surgeon (veterinarian).

Sand colic

If a horse takes in large amounts of sand or silt whilst drinking, or grazing, as happens when the grazing on such soils is poor, then these materials tend to pass along the alimentary tract as far as the caecum. Here they accumulate until eventually the whole caecum becomes impacted. This impaction is particularly difficult to treat by medical means, and surgery may be the only hope.

Sand colic caused by drinking from streams with sandy beds should be avoided by the provision of another satisfactory drinking source, and the discouragement of drinking from the stream. Sand colic is more common in the USA than in Britain because more natural sources of water are used for horses to drink from.

Acute colic

Most cases of acute colic are spasmodic in character. The acute pain lasts for a period of between 10 and 60 minutes, and then there is a period of apparent relief before another period of pain starts. During the spasm the pain may cause the horse to throw himself to the ground and roll violently whilst kicking at his abdomen. Even during the periods of comparative relief, if the horse has simple indigestion with gas pains, listening to the abdomen with a stethoscope will reveal that there are still excessive bowel movements. The majority of these cases have a nervous origin. Perhaps there has been some interruption of the horse's normal routine (they are great creatures of habit), or perhaps something has startled him. Although the reason may not be obvious, something as insignificant as that can be the sole cause of a major problem.

Horse owners are often in a quandary as to what their attitude should be towards a horse with colic. I would suggest that you watch the horse closely, and:

If the pain is not too severe and then subsides, continue watching for an hour before pronouncing the horse recovered.

If the mild pain does not subside, or if it reoccurs, seek veterinary advice.

If the pain is severe, contact your veterinary surgeon (veterinarian) immediately. While you are awaiting his arrival you may walk the horse around to discourage him from throwing himself down and possibly injuring himself. Do not walk a horse out if he is still trying to throw himself down.

Treatment of acute colic should relieve the pain and restore normal bowel movements. Morphine was the first effective drug used in horses with colic. The doses used were sometimes enormous! We now have modern derivatives of morphine available which are just as effective at relieving pain but without the side effects of morphine. Merely treating the pain does not, however, treat the whole problem although when the horse is able to relax his bowel movements may well improve. Spasmolytic agents do actually relax the bowels and allow the normal rhythm to return. The use of these two types of drug has revolutionized the treatment of colic, which is no longer as serious a problem as it used to be when horses in prolonged acute pain caused themselves all kinds of serious injuries.

In some cases, unfortunately, the acute pain is not spasmodic but continuous. This occurs when there is some serious physical change in the bowels. Associated with this continuous pain the horse usually runs a fever and has an increasingly rapid heart rate. The sort of internal changes which can occur include the longitudinal twisting of a section of the bowel, or the pushing of a loop of bowel through a small hole in the supporting membranes so that it becomes strangulated. Obviously no amount of drugs is going to correct this sort of physical displacement. A few cases will right themselves, but in the majority of cases the bowel damage can result in such a degree of shock that the horse will die.

At least that was the case until the late 1960s. Since that time, however, more and more horses suffering from acute colic have undergone successful abdominal surgery to remove the cause of the pain. I must make it clear that no veterinary surgeon (veterinarian) would suggest abdominal surgery in a shocked horse unless it was absolutely necessary, but when the other alternatives are euthanasia or certain death then surgery may be the horse's only hope. If surgery is to be successful it must not be too long delayed. It is no use either owner or veterinary surgeon (veterinarian) delaying surgery until the horse has deteriorated even more, and expecting to have the same chances of success. One group of German practitioners operating on nearly 100 horses with acute colic every year has reported success rates of between 66% and 85%, when surgery is done before shock becomes advanced, so this treatment is not just a forlorn hope.

LAMINITIS (FOUNDER)

Some horse owners may be a little surprised to see laminitis, or founder, included as a feeding problem, rather than as, say, a foot problem. I have done this in order to emphasize that this painful problem in the foot is so often a by-product of mistakes made over feed intake.

Laminitis can also occur following severe infections, drug reactions, and exhaustion. By far the majority of cases, however, arise from too much rich feed given to normal horses, or ordinary amounts of customary feeds given to certain ponies, especially those showing hard patchy fat lumped in the crest of the neck, along the tops of the ribs, and around the tail.

As far as the average horse owner is concerned, laminitis is an extremely painful condition affecting any number of the horse's feet. Early on, there is no increased heat in the feet, as has so often been suggested. Only days later, when inflammation is well developed, do the hooves feel notably warm. Affected animals are said to walk like a cat on a hot tin roof. In severe cases they may not be willing to walk at all, no matter what methods you use to stimulate them.

Rotation of the pedal bone in laminitis.

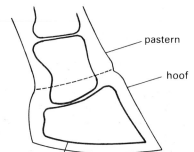

bearing surface of normal pedal bone parallel to sole of hoof

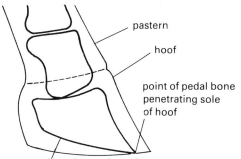

point of pedal bone penetrating sole of hoof

rotated bearing surface of bone

Following some excellent research work in America, veterinary surgeons now look on laminitis in a completely different way.

Laminitis is rather like stomach migraine in human beings. The horse fills his stomach with too much carbohydrate. Among the side-effects which then occur is the dilation of certain blood vessels. If these blood vessels are unable to dilate, as in the foot where they are surrounded by horn, then pain results, but this is a by-product of the original 'overfeeding' not the main feature of the ailment. It has been possible to study laminitis in depth because by passing a stomach tube and administering large amounts of carbohydrates, it is possible to produce laminitis at will in ponies.

Although horse owners do not go around consciously overfeeding their animals with carbohydrates, they do expose them to the attractions of lush pastures. The leaf part of grasses and clover is very rich in carbohydrate. Feeding large quantities of cereals or horse nuts prior to an event is another potentially dangerous source of high carbohydrate concentrations in the stomach. One of the first, though unseen, symptoms of laminitis is a marked slowing of the movement of food down the whole alimentary tract. This aggravates everything, because it means that the carbohydrate food stays in the stomach even longer. When a horse or pony does find a good patch of lush grazing, he does not need to move around a great deal to eat his fill, and so the circulation in the foot slows even further. Indeed laminitis, like so many diseases, is an example of a balance being upset. Feeding too much carbohydrate will tip the balance even if exercise is normal. Alternately if a horse fails to receive adequate exercise, he may suffer from laminitis on a quite average diet. Some ponies definitely have an underlying susceptibility to the condition, and only need a slight tip in the balance before they show symptoms.

I hope it is now clear why the initial treatment of laminitis should aim at emptying the alimentary tract and removing the food which is the initial cause of the problem. Bran mashes, possibly containing some epsom salts, may be sufficient for this purpose in mild cases. In more acute cases your veterinary surgeon may have to administer a purgative by stomach tube.

There are various ways of relieving the pain in the horse's feet. Exercise is essential, no matter how unwilling to move the animal may be. This is definitely a case where you must be cruel to be kind. It might even be necessary to use local anaesthetics in order to block the pain in the feet and get the circulation moving again with exercise. Opinions vary as to how important the frog of the horse's foot is in stimulating circulation. Some people think it is vital to have the frog in firm contact with the ground when the weight is on the foot because this acts as a pumping mechanism. Other people are not convinced that frog pressure has any significant effect. I prefer to be safe, and like to ensure that horses with laminitis are putting pressure on their frogs when walking.

Anti-inflammatory drugs such as the corticosteroids or the non-steroidal anti-inflammatory agents are very useful for counteracting the effects of laminitis in both the body and the feet. Hosing the horse's feet, or standing him in a stream, will cool the feet and cause constriction of some of the blood vessels.

Despite all these efforts, some cases of laminitis become chronic, with permanent changes in the foot. The pedal bone in the foot can rotate so that instead of the flat surface of the bone resting on the sensitive laminae of the sole, the pointed 'toe' of the bone does so. If X-rays show that such changes have taken place, it is very serious. Altering the angle of the whole hoof by trimming etc. may relieve the pressure, but if the changes are too great, euthanasia may be necessary.

Horses which suffer from laminitis usually produce poor and crumbling horn. This is due to a deficiency in the body of a vital substance, D.L. methionine, which acts as a bridge to hold the horn molecules together. This poor horn may be laid down in the walls, giving the hoof wall a ringed appearance (so beware of buying an animal with hooves such as this), or it may be laid down in the sole of the hoof. Feeding extra D.L. methionine in the horse's food will help to ensure that future horn is of better quality, but cannot cause any improvement in existing faulty horn.

THE 'HORSE SICK' PASTURE

The term 'horse sick' has a variety of meanings. It may mean simply that the pasture has been overgrazed to the point where the grass can no longer recover and grow again. This is increasingly the case in suburban areas, where more and more people are keeping horses and ponies on less and less land. In Britain the British Horse Society has had to bring out a special booklet with the self-explanatory title *Horses & Ponies on small areas* to encounter this problem.

'Horse sick' may refer to the type of herbage left following many years of selective equine grazing. Horses leave up to half the pasture as a rough, ungrazed area for dunging etc. Weeds can easily colonize these areas without being checked by grazing, and will strangle the grasses.

Finally the term 'horse sick' may mean that there are too many worm eggs on the pasture as a result of grazing relatively large numbers of horses without any proper worm prevention measures. Obviously if the worm challenge is too great, no horse will be able to thrive. Resting the pasture for several years, preferably whilst still allowing grazing by cattle or sheep, may be sufficient to solve the problem where ploughing and 'crop rotation' is impossible. In more borderline cases regular worming at four to six week intervals throughout the year will, over the space of a couple of years, reduce the problem to more manageable proportions.

5 Diseases of the heart and lungs

The diseases of the heart and lungs are intrinsically linked together. Air enters the lungs in order to come into intimate contact with the fine blood vessels through which the body will absorb oxygen and release its waste carbon dioxide. Circulation through the blood vessels of the lung is powered by the right side of the heart, and only when it has been around this system is the blood pumped out into the general circulation by the left side of the heart. Any ailment which affects one part of the heart/lung complex puts a corresponding strain on the other part, because the horse tries to maintain adequate oxygen levels throughout his body no matter how much effort is needed to provide them.

Respiratory obstructions

The respiratory system consists of the nasal chambers or sinuses, the larynx or voice box, the trachea or windpipe and the lungs. An obstruction of any one of these parts, no matter how slight, will reduce the amount of oxygen available for the blood.

LARYNGEAL OBSTRUCTIONS
Although very occasional physical obstructions are found in the nasal chambers, the first major site of respiratory obstruction is the larynx. When the passage of air through this semi-rigid 'box' is obstructed, turbulence develops which gives rise to a roaring noise. Now 'roaring' is well known as a respiratory defect, although surprisingly few horse owners could define it accurately. It is not sufficient to say that it is a noise made when the horse is exercised strongly, because every horse in the world makes a noise of some kind when he breathes out during cantering or galloping. Only if a horse makes two noises, i.e. if he makes an abnormal noise on inspiration (breathing in) as well as the normal noise on expiration (breathing out), should the horse be said to be a roarer. You can tell which noise is which quite readily because at such fast paces the horse breathes out when the leading foreleg hits the ground.

It is a common fallacy that a horse will only 'roar' if he has a paralysed vocal chord, but this is not the case. Swollen and inflamed areas in the pharynx, which is the chamber where the mouth, nasal chambers, oesophagus and larynx all meet, are but one of several other causes of roaring. Diagnosis of the cause (which must obviously precede any decision on treatment) can only be accurately made by using an endoscope to look directly at the horse's larynx.

Laryngeal paralysis, or laryngeal hemiplegia, is a paralysis of the left vocal chord in the horse's larynx. Normally these vocal chords lie partially across the larynx when the horse is not under any strain and are pulled aside by the laryngeal muscles during fast exercise. In a horse with laryngeal paralysis, the left vocal chord is not pulled out of the way during fast exercise and there is some obstruction of the air flow through the larynx. The underlying cause of this failure is the degeneration of a long nerve which stretches all the way from the horse's brain down his neck into his chest and then back up to the

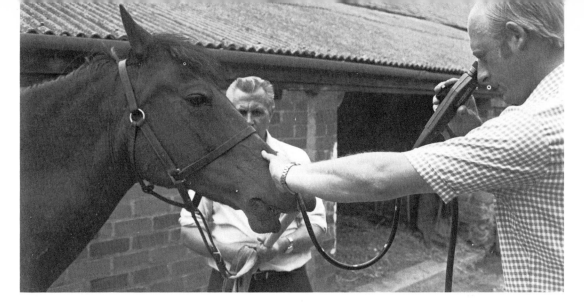

small muscle which should pull the left chord out of the way. For various reasons, not all of which are fully understood, it is always the left nerve/muscle/vocal chord which is affected.

The condition usually affects large horses, and its incidence can be as high as 50% in horses over 17hh. It is, however, only of clinical importance when it limits a horse's performance. So it is worth remembering that not only is every roarer not suffering from laryngeal paralysis, but not every roarer needs treatment. If a horse performs well, you must ask yourself what you hope to achieve from treatment.

Just as roaring is a well known abnormality, the Hobday operation is a well known treatment for this condition. The operation consists of removing the lining of the left laryngeal ventricle, a cavity which lies behind the vocal chord. It was always hoped that the scar tissue formed during healing would pull the vocal chord outwards, and so allow easier passage of air through the larynx. The use of the endoscope has shown that in most cases there is little or no effect on the position of the vocal chord. Because the scar tissue fills up and obliterates the ventricle, it will often (but not always) decrease the air turbulence and the resultant roaring, but the airway is still not completely open at fast exercise.

Although this may sound like heresy to some people who have had horses hobdayed, we must remember that Professor Hobday himself reckoned that only about 20% of horses he operated on were sufficiently successful to 'pass the average hunting man without comment'. It has

Using an endoscope to examine a horse's larynx: by passing a flexible tube up a horse's nostril the vet (veterinarian) can look directly up the larynx. The majority of horses will allow this procedure to be carried out with just a twitch as a restraint.

The horse's larynx (voice box) seen through an endoscope.

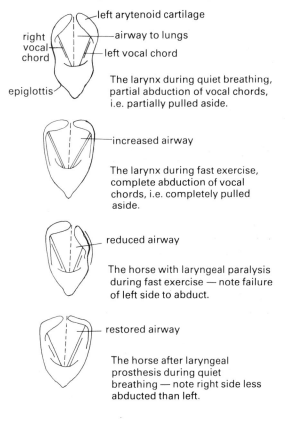

left arytenoid cartilage

right vocal chord

airway to lungs

left vocal chord

epiglottis

The larynx during quiet breathing, partial abduction of vocal chords, i.e. partially pulled aside.

increased airway

The larynx during fast exercise, complete abduction of vocal chords, i.e. completely pulled aside.

reduced airway

The horse with laryngeal paralysis during fast exercise — note failure of left side to abduct.

restored airway

The horse after laryngeal prosthesis during quiet breathing — note right side less abducted than left.

also been pointed out that owners are often reluctant to work a 'roarer' fully, and so do not get the horse properly fit. After an operation, however, they feel safe to do so and find that the fit horse (with or without any improvement in his larynx) is better than he was before.

It is possible to improve the air flow through the larynx surgically. This is done by using a prosthesis, which is an artificial replacement for a faulty part of the body. An elastic prosthesis can be inserted which replaces the muscles which are failing to pull the left vocal chord out of the way at exercise. The result of this rather intricate operation is that the horse has the left vocal chord held out of the way permanently, whether at rest or fast exercise. This results in quiet and efficient breathing even at fast exercise.

So I would suggest that:

1 Horses which roar but do not have laryngeal paralysis when examined with an endoscope should not be operated on.
2 Horses which have laryngeal paralysis but are performing satisfactorily should not be operated on.
3 Horses which have laryngeal paralysis and show some distress when exercised may benefit from a Hobday operation.
4 Horses with laryngeal paralysis which show marked distress when exercised or which are required to compete at a reasonably high level may benefit most from a prosthesis operation.

Before leaving the larynx, I would like to mention the condition known as 'tongue swallowing'. This is a gurgling noise some horses make when galloping really flat out, and it is accompanied by an abrupt loss of performance. What happens is that the muscles of the neck pull the larynx out of the socket where it joins the pharynx. This obviously interferes with the air flow into the larynx, with dramatic results. As soon as the pressure is off the horse because it has slowed down, the larynx returns to its normal position and the noise vanishes. Strapping the tongue down so that the whole tongue/larynx mechanism cannot be pulled backwards may give some improvement, but the real cure lies in surgically removing part of the muscles which pull the larynx out of position.

OBSTRUCTIVE LUNG DISEASE, CHRONIC OBSTRUCTIVE PULMONARY DISEASE (C.O.P.D.)

The other major site for obstruction of the airway is in the lungs. The obstruction in this case is due to two factors. Firstly increased amounts of really thick viscous mucus may block some of the small bronchioles or airways in the lungs.

Secondly the muscles surrounding the bronchioles go into a spasm, and this bronchospasm, as it is called, dramatically reduces the cross-sectional area of the airway.

Not surprisingly, horses which suffer from such chronic obstructive pulmonary disease (C.O.P.D.) are not capable of full work. Even at

The effects of bronchospasm: cross-section of one of the tiny bronchioles in the lung.

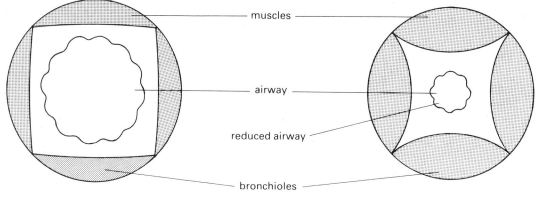

muscles

airway

reduced airway

bronchioles

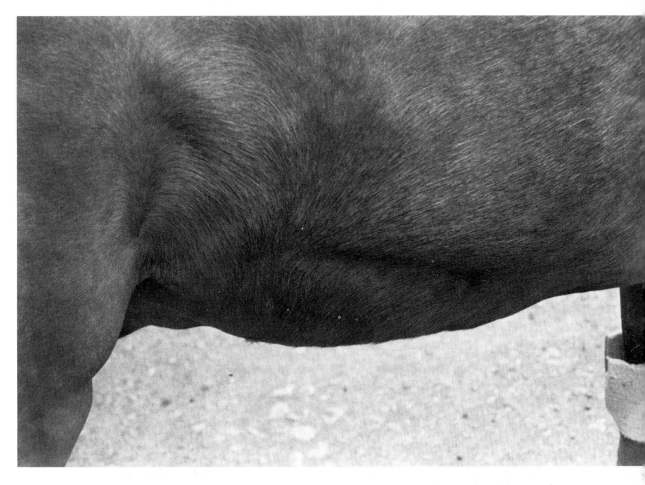

rest their expiration will appear broken into two parts (hence the old name of 'broken wind') because although the air appears to be able to enter the lungs normally, the usual elastic recoil of the lungs is not sufficiently powerful to push the air out again past this obstruction. As a result the horse has to push forcefully with the muscles of his thorax and abdomen in order to empty the lungs. This muscular effort has given rise to another traditional name for this condition, 'heaves'. Over a long period the muscles involved may become over-developed, and it is possible to see a 'heave line' between them along the lower belly.

C.O.P.D. is an allergic disease. The horse develops an allergy to the dust and fungal spores which he breathes in from straw bedding, hay etc. When the horse's lung recognises the

Heave line on the abdomen of a horse suffering from C.O.P.D. The muscles become over-developed due to the extra effort needed to breathe out.

presence of such irritants, the allergic reaction results in the release of histamines etc. and the bronchiolar muscles go into a bronchospasm. The horse also starts to cough, which is his basic defence mechanism to remove unwanted objects from his lungs. Finally, as I have already mentioned, an increased amount of thickened mucus is formed and some of this may show as a nasal discharge. You will notice that I have not mentioned emphysema, which is the permanent breakdown of lung tissue. This is because such extreme damage is now known to be extremely rare, and not a usual accompaniment of C.O.P.D.

The first stage of treating C.O.P.D. is obviously to remove the cause of the allergy. So instead of the dusty air normally found in stables, you must provide clean fresh air. This means that there must be good ventilation for the stable, with a relatively large air volume per horse. It means that the stable should be clean and dust free. It means that no straw should be used for bedding, nor should straw be used or kept in the same airspace. It means that if hay is fed it should be well soaked, but that ideally complete horse nuts (feed pellets in USA) should be substituted. The ideal stable for a C.O.P.D. horse is an open field.

In many cases fresh air therapy will result in the horse apparently returning to normal, although you must always remember that if his lungs are exposed to the irritants at some later date, e.g. because the horse is transported in a horsebox (horse van) which has straw bedding, then the symptoms will return. In other cases the recovery will be very slow, perhaps because

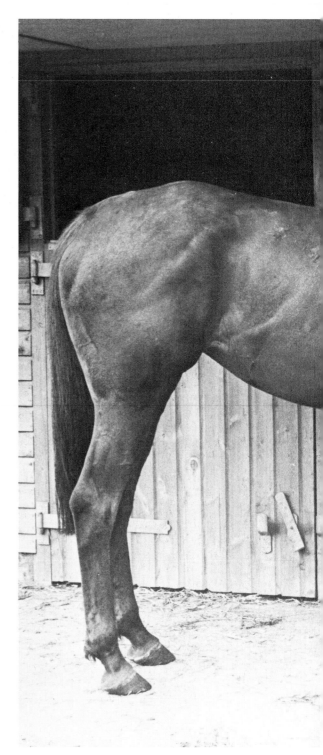

Symptoms of C.O.P.D. (broken wind)

Cough

Decreased performance

Broken wind

Nose bleeds

Nasal discharge

An electric nebuliser used to administer such drugs as sodium chromoglycate, sold in Britain as Chromovet.

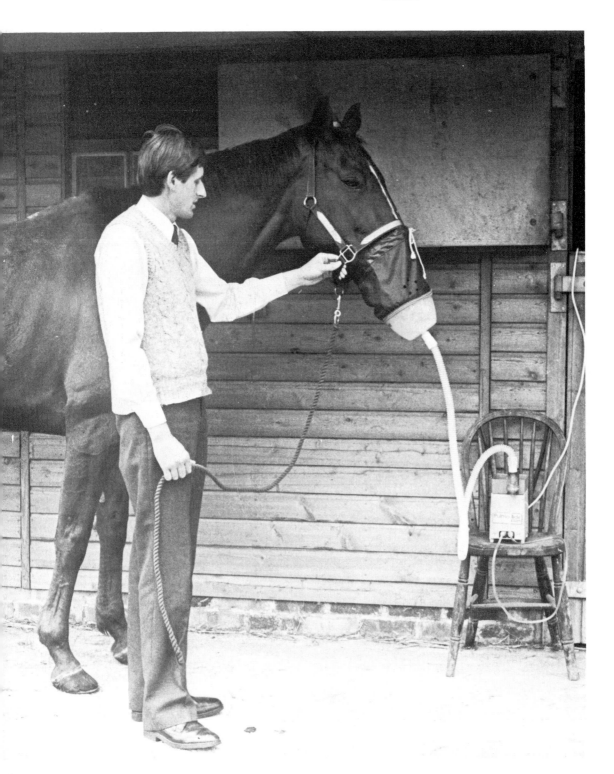

the bronchospasm is too firmly established. The use of bronchodilator drugs such as clenbuterol is very useful here. This is available in Britain and should be shortly in the USA. This drug relaxes the muscles in the bronchioles, enabling the horse to breathe freely. It also thins the mucus and speeds up its removal.

If it really is impossible to provide fresh air for a horse with C.O.P.D. then it is possible, following treatment with bronchodilators etc., to use drugs to inhibit the whole allergic reaction. At present this requires the use of an electric nebuliser to administer the drug, so it is not the ideal method.

The emphasis in the treatment of respiratory obstructions is obviously on restoring normal air flow. The diseases tend to be self-limiting, in that the lack of oxygen causes an affected horse to slow down, with the result that he needs less oxygen and so the effect of the obstruction is less important.

Respiratory infections

The relative importance of the various respiratory infections which can affect the horse has changed markedly over the years, and continues to do so. Fifty years ago the most important respiratory disease would have been strangles. During the 1970s it was equine influenza which proved most troublesome, and now that vaccination policies appear to be lessening the effect of equine influenza, we find that the rhino-pneumonitis virus is capable of seriously disrupting equine activities. Glanders was once a scourge throughout the world, but now eradication methods have almost eliminated it. Of course we do not know what the future will bring; perhaps diseases such as equine viral arteritis (see page 50) will spread to Britain, where at present they are unknown. One thing which is certain is that modern international transport of horses will enable respiratory and other diseases to spread much more rapidly than they have in the past.

STRANGLES (SOMETIMES KNOWN AS 'DISTEMPER' IN USA)
Strangles is a bacterial disease, the bacteria responsible being called Streptococcus equi. It affects young animals especially, and so is commonest when groups of young horses are gathered together after weaning or for sales purposes. There is usually a very high temperature, up to 41°C (106°F), and a thick nasal discharge. The bacteria becomes lodged in the lymph glands around the head and elsewhere. In most cases these glands become very swollen, hot and painful, ultimately bursting and releasing thick pus.

In some parts of the world a vaccine is available to protect horses against strangles. The vaccine, which is not without side-effects, is not available in Britain. Treatment with antibiotics, usually penicillin, is very successful and has drastically reduced the importance of this disease. Treatment which is too brief (less than 7 days) may drive the organism 'underground', only to reappear as a more sinister disease of the chest or abdomen.

EQUINE INFLUENZA
Although there are two distinct strains of equine influenza virus (in contrast to the situation in man where there are hundreds of strains) the symptoms are basically common to both the type one (Prague) strain and the type two (Miami) strain. Infected horses give a frequent dry cough and go off their food. They run a temperature of 40°C (104°F) and have a clear nasal discharge.

The influenza virus is extremely contagious and spreads very rapidly within a group of susceptible horses. Infected horses are capable of passing the virus on to other animals even before any clinical symptoms appear, so isolation of coughing horses is not as successful a means of controlling the spread of the disease as one would have hoped. The incubation period is between three and ten days, and it tends to shorten as an outbreak of flu gains strength. Of course the very act of coughing helps the spread of the disease because the viruses are coughed out into the atmosphere.

Coughing may persist for three or four weeks after the infection. Because of the effect of the virus on the heart and lung tissue, horses which have suffered from equine flu must have at least six weeks complete rest before starting exercise again. Failure to allow this convalescent period may result in permanent heart and lung damage.

Foals are especially at risk to the type one virus because they cannot develop any immunity until they are about three months old. Any protection must come from the colostrum, or first milk, which they obtain from their mothers during the first 12 hours of life.

There are no drugs available which will cure equine flu by killing the viruses. Treatment must instead concentrate on relieving some of the symptoms of the disease. Cough syrups, powders and electuaries are widely used but have little effect on the course of the disease. In any case the cough is basically a protective mechanism to free the lungs of excess mucous, so it is not necessarily an undesirable symptom. Broncho-dilators such as clenbuterol will speed up removal of mucous and reverse the broncho-spasm which occurs in infections like this just as readily as it does in C.O.P.D. In some cases the mucous becomes infected with secondary bacteria. When this happens the nasal discharge becomes thick and pussy, whilst the fever continues for even longer. Treatment with antibiotics, either orally or by injection, is then necessary.

Equine flu is usually an epidemic disease. The only hope of containing it when an outbreak occurs is by vaccination. The vaccines available protect against both strains of virus involved. Even vaccinated horses may cough mildly for a day or two when exposed to the disease, but generally the vaccines are very effective. The higher the proportion of vaccinated horses in a stable yard, the more effective the vaccine will be.

The racing authorities of Britain, Ireland and France have agreed a common vaccination policy, which is also now being adopted by most non-racing interests such as show and sales directors. The basic requirement is for two primary injections of vaccine separated by between three and twelve weeks. These are then followed by annual booster vaccinations. There is evidence, however, that the immunity produced by the primary course of injections does not last a full twelve months. For this reason it is being suggested that the first booster should be given five to seven months after the primary course, with annual boosters thereafter. The racing authorities are requiring this course to be followed for all horses born after January 1st 1980. Brood mares should have their boosters about three or four weeks before foaling, so that the maximum possible level of immunity is available to the foal in the colostrum.

RHINOPNEUMONITIS

Rhinopneumonitis is another viral disease which involves two distinct strains of virus, in this case a Herpes virus. Type one rhinopneumonitis causes abortion in pregnant mares. The mares may show a slight nasal discharge initially and then within a week or so they abort or give birth to a weak premature foal. The disease is so infectious that within three or four weeks most of the other pregnant mares which have been in even slight contact will also abort. These abortion storms can create havoc when expensive brood mares are kept together in large numbers, as they are in America.

The type two rhinopneumonitis virus causes respiratory symptoms, especially in young horses. Although of comparatively little importance in America, this virus is responsible for nearly 50% of respiratory infections in British racing stables. Infected horses have a fever and a clear nasal discharge. The glands of the head and neck are often swollen. Affected horses not only fail to perform as well as they did prior to infection, in some cases this loss of performance continues for three or four months. Immunity following the clinical disease is short lived and horses may succumb to infection again in as little as three months.

As with equine influenza, there is no cure for rhinopneumonitis, although symptomatic treatment of the respiratory disease is of value. Stringent hygiene is essential on any stud where a rhinopneumonitis abortion occurs. No horses should be moved from the premises until well after everything has returned to normal, because even horses which do not succumb to the disease may pass it on to other, more susceptible, horses.

There are two types of vaccine available against rhinopneumonitis abortion. The first vaccines developed were live vaccines. These are very effective and stimulate immunity rapidly but there is a definite risk of the live virus involved causing a low level of abortions in its own right. More recently a dead vaccine has been developed. As the virus here has been killed, there is no risk of vaccination causing abortion. Multiple injections are, however, necessary during pregnancy before full protection is achieved.

There are no vaccines available specifically for the type two virus. The pattern of the disease is, however, changing all the time and an increasing number of outbreaks of respiratory disease are now being blamed on the type one abortion strain. It remains to be seen whether vaccination against this strain will protect against these and other respiratory outbreaks.

EQUINE VIRAL ARTERITIS

In some parts of the world another viral disease, viral arteritis, is important as a cause of both respiratory symptoms and abortion. Following an incubation period of a week or less, infected horses have a fever with conjunctivitis (which is why the disease is sometimes called 'Pink eye'). The horses have a nasal discharge.

The symptoms are due to damage to the walls of the arteries, especially those which 'feed' the respiratory and reproductive tracts. Very young and very old horses are particularly susceptible. There are no treatments and no vaccines available but luckily mortality is low.

Blood disorders

It is important to appreciate that blood is not just a red liquid. It consists of a pale straw-coloured fluid which is called the plasma, in which are suspended large numbers of microscopic cells. The plasma is the horse's reservoir of fluid and also transports various soluble substances such as proteins, carbohydrates etc. from one part of the body to another. The blood cells form two main groups depending on their colour when viewed under the microscope. The red cells are concerned with transporting oxygen from the lungs where it is in a high concentration, to the various body tissues which need it. The white cells have a variety of functions, but are basically involved in the various defensive mechanisms of the body. The total blood volume of a horse is about 30 litres/9 gallons in USA/6½ gallons in Britain.

Diseases affecting the red cells

The red blood cells of mammals such as the horse are unique among the body's cells because they have no nuclei. They contain a pigment called haemoglobin which has the ability to combine with oxygen when this is readily available and transport this oxygen around the circulatory system until an area is reached where oxygen levels are low. The oxygen is then released, and its place taken by the carbon dioxide which abounds as a waste product of all bodily functions.

The resting horse stores large numbers of blood cells in its spleen. Any slight excitement, including exercise, results in some of these stored cells being squeezed out into the general circulation. If it is necessary to take a blood sample from a horse, which is usually done via the jugular vein in the neck, it is important that the sample is taken from a quiet resting horse, or a falsely high red cell count may be obtained. A normal resting horse has between 8,000,000 and 12,000,000 red blood cells in every cubic millilitre of blood, but these levels can rise by as much as a third following even gentle trotting exercise.

ANAEMIA ✓

Anaemia is a shortage of haemoglobin in the body. It can arise in several different ways. If a horse is badly cut and loses a great deal of blood, then the number of red blood cells (and hence the amount of haemoglobin) in the body will be low. In this form of anaemia a count of the number of red cells present per millilitre of blood will be low, but each of the remaining red cells will contain a normal amount of haemoglobin. The anaemia will cease to exist as soon as the body replaces the lost red blood cells. It normally takes about three weeks from the earliest stage in manufacturing a red blood cell until the cell is sufficiently mature to function properly in the general circulation. The red blood cells are comparatively short lived because of their lack of nucleus, and so are continually being replaced.

A much smaller blood loss, but occurring over

Blood smear showing the different types of cells usually present

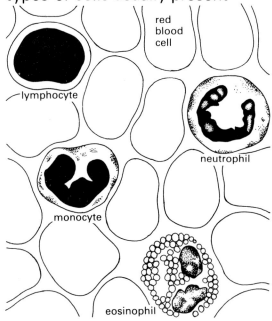

lymphocyte

red blood cell

neutrophil

monocyte

eosinophil

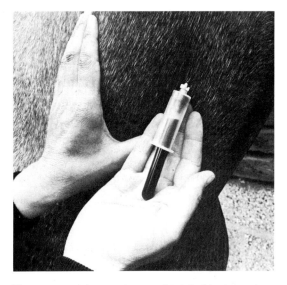

The vacuum syringe system used to take blood samples.

Taking a blood sample from the large jugular vein in a horse's neck.

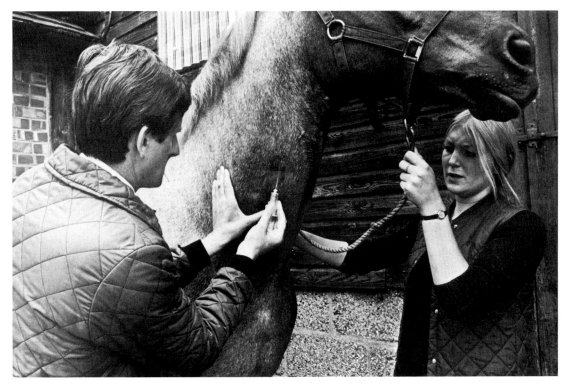

a much longer time, can occur due to parasites. External parasites such as lice and fleas can suck blood, and if these parasites are present in very large numbers then this results in a marked anaemia. Worms can also cause this sort of chronic anaemia.

The red blood cell count may also be due to a rather important vitamin deficiency. The horse needs a vitamin called folic acid for the manufacture of both red and white blood cells. Folic acid is present in quite large amounts in grass and other herbage but when these are made into hay, substantial amounts of the vitamin are lost. Horses which are stabled for long periods without regular access to grazing are often deficient in folic acid, and so are both anaemic (due to a shortage of red blood cells) and have a low white blood cell count. Feeding lucerne (alfalfa) hay, which usually has good folic acid levels, may solve the problem, but failing this high levels of folic acid must be added to the food. In Britain no available food supplement contains sufficient folic acid to treat a deficiency; and the vitamin has to be administered in pure form.

Anaemia due to lack of iron is far less common than horse owners, influenced as they are by advertising for so-called blood tonics and iron supplements, ever imagine. Both grazing and most stable and commercial feeds contain adequate levels of iron, which is necessary as the major constituent of haemoglobin. When there is a deficiency of iron it is usually because stress, such as during a strenuous training programme, has increased the horse's requirements for new red blood cells beyond normal levels, rather than because levels in the diet are lower than normal. The same situation applies to vitamin B12, which occasionally as a result of stress and lack of grazing may become deficient and cause anaemia. Again, high levels of the deficient substances must be fed if they are to have any real effect on the anaemia.

All forms of anaemia have similar symptoms. Except in really severe cases this does not include any discernible effect on the horse's mucous membranes. It is not possible to decide whether a horse needs extra iron or folic acid just because a so-called expert says his membranes 'look pale'. Affected horses are listless and perform poorly. Appetite is often depressed. In some cases anaemia causes a temporary heart murmur, which disappears when the anaemia is cured.

BLOOD TYPING

It is now possible to blood type a horse in a way similar to that used for human beings. This is usually used as a means of checking parentage. Although it is not possible to say 'this horse is the parent of that foal', because of the remote chance of two horses having the same blood type, it is possible to say that 'this horse cannot be the parent of that foal'. In the 1981 Irish stud season, routine blood typing showed that a couple of foals thought to have been sired by one desirable stallion could not possibly have been sired by him.

The first step in typing a horse's blood is to detect the presence or absence of 7 out of the 30 recognised groups of red blood cells. These major groups are the A, C, D, K, P, Q, and U systems. The second part of the typing is done by checking for 8 protein systems which may be present. This is done by placing a drop of blood on to a starch 'jelly' covered plate. When an electric current is passed through the jelly it separates the protein systems by carrying them with the current for varying distances. The various proteins present can then be identified.

Diseases affecting the white cells

There are four main types of white blood cell; neutrophils, monocytes, lymphocytes and eosinophils. The total number of white blood cells is very much less than the number of red blood cells in a horse's blood. A healthy horse will have approximately as many thousands of white blood cells per millilitre of blood as he has millions of red blood cells. Of the four main types of white blood cell about 60% are neutrophils and 40% lymphocytes, with the other cells only present in very small numbers.

The white blood cells are all concerned with the horse maintaining his normal health against outside influences. The eosinophil, for instance, is involved in any allergic responses by the body.

Severe worm infestations often result in a form of allergic reaction to the worms, and so a higher than normal percentage of eosinophils often indicates the presence of large numbers of worms. The other minority white blood cell is the monocyte, which is involved in the horse's reaction to certain chronic types of infection.

The most numerous white blood cell is the neutrophil. This cell's main role is to destroy bacteria. Often this results in the neutrophil itself being destroyed. Indeed, pus is basically a collection of dead bacteria and dead neutrophils. When a horse has been exposed to a bacterial infection he manufactures an increased number of neutrophils, which shows as an increased percentage of these cells in a cell count.

The lymphocyte is more involved in the production of antibodies, the proteins which protect the body against viruses etc. A viral infection is one cause of an increased percentage of lymphocytes.

Diseases affecting blood circulation

Without the heart there is no blood circulation. The heart is a rather unique type of pump. It obtains its energy sources from the very blood which it exists to pump around the body.

It may be more convenient to look on the heart as two separate pumps fixed together side by side. Blood enters the right atrium of the heart from the major vein in the body, the vena cava. At this stage the blood is low in oxygen. From the right side of the heart the blood is pumped to the lungs. Here it passes through increasingly fine blood vessels until eventually the blood is separated from the air in the lungs by only the thickness of one cell. Here the haemoglobin of the blood releases any carbon dioxide which it is carrying and absorbs in its place some of the oxygen which fills the lungs.

The heart and circulation.

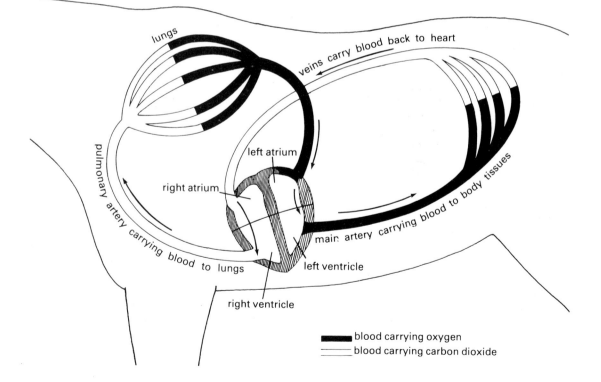

lungs

veins carry blood back to heart

pulmonary artery carrying blood to lungs

left atrium

right atrium

main artery carrying blood to body tissues

left ventricle

right ventricle

blood carrying oxygen
blood carrying carbon dioxide

The fine blood vessels then merge into themselves until they form a single blood vessel again, the pulmonary vein. This oxygen-rich blood then enters the left side of the heart, where the valves and pumps send it on its way around the rest of the body.

It will thus be obvious to you that any defect of the right side of the heart will firstly reduce the blood flow through the lungs, and secondly cause a hold-up in the general circulation. This congestion of the veins returning blood to the heart may become so severe, and the walls of the veins so stretched and porous, that fluid leaks out of the circulation. Hence the finding of dropsy (fluid in the abdomen) or 'filled' legs in some horses with heart trouble. Any defect of the left side of the heart will firstly reduce the blood flow around the body, and secondly cause a hold-up in the circulation of blood through the lungs. Congestion like this in the lungs may give rise to a chronic cough.

When we listen to a horse's heart through a stethoscope we expect to hear two heart sounds. The noise sounds rather like 'lub-dub'. In many normal horses at rest the first sound appears split into two parts, and in others the rhythm is very irregular. These are accepted as normal, but after fast exercise the horse should have regular normal heart sounds. Any abnormality which appears with exercise or which gets worse with exercise is undesirable.

Of course, veterinary surgeons (veterinarians) are not infallible. Just as there are many men walking around in good health years after they were given three months to live, so there are many horses performing successfully after a

Using a stethoscope to listen to a horse's heart.

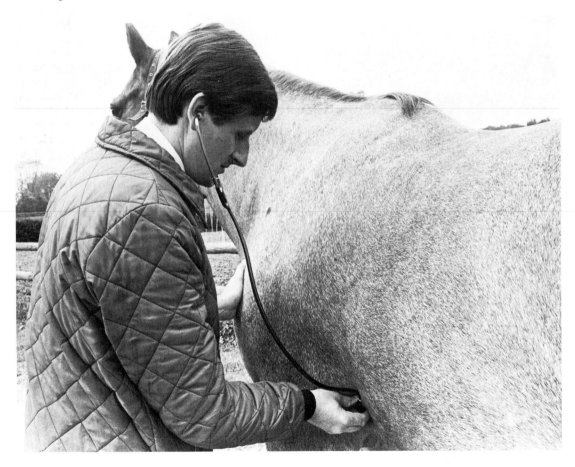

Electrocardiograph trace.

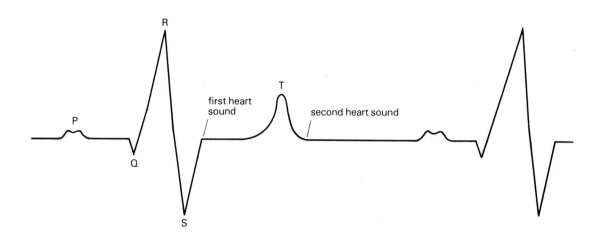

veterinary surgeon (veterinarian) advised someone not to buy the horse because it had a bad heart. All we can do is to make a well-informed judgement. We cannot ignore heart disease, because the risk of serious damage to rider or others should a horse collapse is too great.

Earlier I likened the heart to a pump. The heart sounds we hear are caused by the heart valves closing during the pumping action. Sometimes the valves are unable to close properly, perhaps due to the development of some physical obstruction. This causes marked turbulence in the blood flow through the heart, and just as turbulence in the horse's larynx causes a roaring noise so turbulence in the blood flow through the heart causes a murmuring sound. These heart murmurs reflect a heart abnormality, they are not physical abnormalities themselves.

In addition to listening to a horse's heart for any abnormal heart sounds, it is also possible to carry out an electrocardiograph (E.C.G.) on the horse. This consists of measuring the minute electrical impulses in the heart from various different positions, and recording them in such a way that even minute abnormalities can be measured and studied at leisure.

Circulatory problems would be expected to severely limit a horse's tolerance to exercise, so he could not achieve his full potential. In the long term, severely affected animals are dull and listless, often with oedema of the legs. Congestion arising in the lungs may cause a chronic cough. A crisis, which is really what a 'heart attack' often amounts to, may occur actually at the time when a supreme demand is made on the circulation, e.g. at a fence, but in many cases the horse collapses and dies when it relaxes after the exertion.

Lack of general fitness will be reflected in the functioning of the heart as well as in the other muscles of movement. In the unfit horse the heart muscles become 'flabby' and unable to work at maximum efficiency, so you must avoid asking too much of your horse in these circumstances. In ensuring that adequate fuel is available for the muscles, vitamin E and selenium are very important. These two substances act in tandem, and both must be available. In some areas there is a soil deficiency of selenium, which causes problems in animals out at grazing. Extra vitamin E and selenium can be given to the horse either by injection or as a food supplement.

6 Diseases of movement

Diagnosis of lameness

It would seem that there are almost as many ideas as to what constitutes lameness as there are weeks in the year. One horse owner considers his horse to be lame if he shortens his stride slightly on one leg. Another owner says his horse 'is a bit lame' when in fact he is scarcely able to walk. I would suggest that a working definition of a lame horse might be one that suffers sufficient discomfort that he is unable to keep his body moving smoothly and level at the trot.

If you suspect that a horse is feeling pain when he moves, then you obviously want to know which leg it is which is causing the problem. You can only do this by observing the horse at paces which involve him putting an equal weight on each leg for an equal length of time. For practical purposes this means watching the horse at the walk and trot. Even then the walk involves so little strain and concussion on the individual legs, that severe pain is usually necessary before a horse is seen to be lame at the walk.

Horse owners are often amazed that horses which trot quite unevenly are able to canter apparently normally. This does not mean that the condition is not very severe, it merely means that because the canter does not involve each leg in turn being subjected to the same strain, our eyes are quite incapable of distinguishing the deviation from normal.

So in order to examine a horse to see if he is lame, have the horse led away from you in a straight line, turned and then walked back. This is something which you cannot do yourself; it is impossible to both lead the horse and assess whether or not he is lame. Make sure that whoever is leading the horse does not hold tightly onto his head, but leaves about 50 cm/ 20 in of loose rein. After you have seen the horse walk, and had a chance to become familiar with his action etc., have him trotted straight away from you and then back, on a hard level surface.

When a horse has to use a leg which hurts, he quite sensibly tries to minimize the pain by putting more weight on his good leg, and taking weight off his bad leg. So if the left front leg hurts, the horse will put more weight on the right front leg; if the right hind leg hurts, the horse will put more weight on the left hind leg. The horse cannot place extra weight on a leg without disturbing the level carriage of the body. So when a foreleg has extra weight placed on it, the head sinks down slightly, or nods. When a hind leg has extra weight on it, the rump sinks down slightly. When you trot a horse up to look for any lameness, you actually look not for the bad leg, but for the good leg. As soon as you know which is the good leg which is bearing the extra weight, you then immediately know which is the lame leg.

I must stress that when a horse is trotted away from you, you look only at the rump. If it 'sinks' regularly, then the leg which is hitting the ground at that time is the sound leg, and the horse is lame on the opposite hind leg. When the horse is trotted towards you, look only at his head. The head sinks on the sound leg, and the horse is lame on the opposite fore leg. Do not make the usual mistake of thinking that the horse 'nods' on the lame leg. If you are in doubt as to whether a horse is 'sinking' or not, it may help you to listen carefully to the noise of the horse's hooves as he moves. The normal trot has a perfectly even rhythm. If it is not a regular rhythm then the horse may well be lame.

Of course there can be complications. If a horse is lame on both forelegs, or both hind legs, he may well appear almost sound at the trot. Sometimes when a horse is lame on one leg it will also appear to be lame on the diagonally opposite leg or on the other leg on the same side. You should not expect to be as expert at diagnosing lameness as an experienced veterinary surgeon (veterinarian), but it is a good idea to watch carefully whenever a lame horse is trotted up because this is definitely an area where practice makes perfect.

Diseases of the foot

Having decided on which leg the horse is lame, then remember that almost certainly the problem lies in the foot. Although horse owners show a marked reluctance to admit the fact, 80% – 90% of all lamenesses are in the foot. This is one of the main reasons for the saying 'no foot, no horse'. Unfortunately, we cannot see or feel what is going on in the foot because of the hard

Anatomy of the foot.

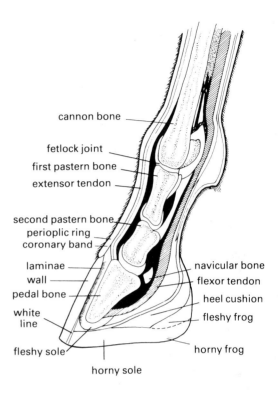

cannon bone

fetlock joint

first pastern bone

extensor tendon

second pastern bone
perioplic ring
coronary band

laminae
wall
pedal bone
white line

fleshy sole

navicular bone
flexor tendon
heel cushion
fleshy frog

horny frog

horny sole

covering of the hoof. Confirmation that the problem lies in the foot may be obtained by putting strong pressure on various parts of the hoof with a hoof tester. If there is any doubt at all as to whether the cause of the lameness is in the foot somewhere or higher up the leg, your veterinary surgeon (veterinarian) will carry out a nerve block. This technique involves injecting a local anaesthetic over the two main nerve branches (one on each side of the leg) which supply the foot. The horse can then no longer feel any pain, or indeed any sensation at all, in the foot. So if a horse goes sound after this nerve block, then the cause of the lameness is in the foot; but if the horse is still lame then you must look with nerve blocks higher up for the source of the problem. Radiography, or the taking of X-ray pictures of the bones, is another specialist technique which it is often necessary to employ when investigating lameness problems.

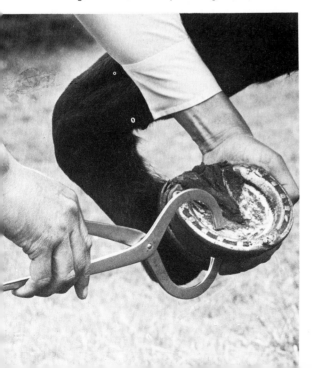

Examining a horse's foot for pain using a hoof tester.

NAVICULAR DISEASE

Navicular disease is a chronic lameness caused by the decay of areas in the navicular bone, which is a small bone lying behind the joint between the pedal bone and the second phalanx.

For some reason which we do not yet understand, some of the tiny blood vessels which supply the navicular bone become blocked by blood clots. Normally all that would happen is that the body would form new blood vessels to supply the affected area, but in certain horses these replacement vessels clot almost as soon as they are formed. The end result is decay of those areas of the bone which are no longer receiving sufficient blood supply.

Navicular disease usually affects the front feet more than the hind feet. It is also more common in horses of eight years of age and over. Often it causes a periodic lameness, i.e the horse may appear lame one day but not the next. In the early stages of the disease the lameness often wears off with exercise, only to return when the horse has stood still for a period of time. Affected feet are often said to become contracted and box-like, although whether this is a predisposing cause of the disease or a result of it is not certain.

Although navicular disease has been recognised for decades, initially there was no treatment available. Neurectomy, the surgical cutting of the nerves supplying the foot, in order that the horse would no longer feel any pain, was

the first attempt to overcome the problem. Unfortunately the severed nerves tend to regrow and re-unite, so that the pain returns. In addition, depriving the horse's foot of a nerve supply may make the horse more prone to injury because he will not receive complete information about what is happening whilst the foot is on the ground bearing the weight of the body.

During the last thirty or forty years, navicular disease has often been 'treated' by the use of anti-inflammatory drugs such as phenylbutazone. These drugs are often able to take away the pain associated with navicular disease, and enable the horse to return to work. It is important to realize, however, that neither neurectomy nor the use of anti-inflammatory drugs has any effect on the degenerating bone in the horse's foot. If the horse continues to work, the bone will continue to deteriorate even if this is no longer obvious to the horse owner.

It is now possible to treat navicular disease by using an anticoagulant. The drug used is warfarin, which is also widely used as a rat poison. The horse is given the warfarin in special tablet form in its feed every day (and it is important that he should not miss a single day's treatment). At the same time blood tests determine the horse's blood 'clotting time', which is the time the blood takes to clot when left to stand.

The aim is to vary the clotting time until it is approximately 30% longer than the pre-treatment time. The result is that when the horse attempts to form new blood vessels in the navicular bone, they no longer become blocked by blood clots. The new blood supply revitalizes the bone, and the pain and lameness gradually disappear. Results from all over the world indicate that approximately 75% of horses treated in this way return to work.

FOOT FRACTURES

One of the greatest Irish racehorses of recent times, who really gripped the imagination of the general public, was the Duchess of Westminster's Arkle. His spectacular steeplechasing career was brought to an end when he fractured a pedal bone, and this focused attention on the problem of fractures in the horse.

Fractures of the pedal bone obviously require

An X-ray of the foot of a horse with navicular disease. Arrows indicate the decaying areas of bone.

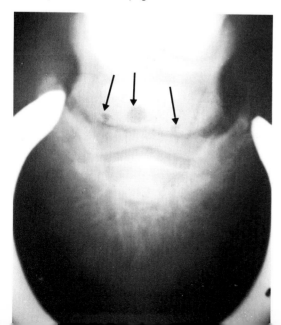

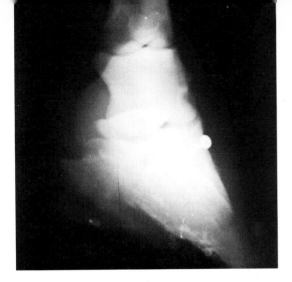

An X-ray of a fractured pedal bone showing the screw in position.

the taking of radiographs if we are to determine precisely what has happened. I mention them here, not because they are a common problem, but to make the point that not all horses with a very acutely painful foot have a fracture, and conversely a horse may appear to have a more chronic type of lameness and yet still actually have a fractured pedal bone. Only reliable radiographs will provide the vital information needed to prove or disprove a diagnosis.

Treatment of pedal bone fractures may be possible purely by a long period of rest, using the hoof as a splint. In some fracture cases, one or more stainless steel screws are inserted into the bone in order to hold the fractured bone together while healing takes place.

PUS IN THE FOOT

The commonest foot problem is probably pus in the foot. This can be the result of a nail, stone, etc. penetrating the sole of the foot, or possibly a crack in the foot wall allowing the entry of infection. Once the infection reaches the rich venous plexus underneath the horn, it multiplies rapidly. The hoof cannot expand to accommodate the resulting pus, and the result is pain and lameness.

Although antibiotics are valuable in killing off the active infection, the lameness will not go until the pressure has been removed by draining the pus. This requires your veterinary surgeon (veterinarian) or farrier to cut an adequate drainage hole from the outside of the hoof down to the very centre of the infection. After this it is up to you to draw out any remaining pus by poulticing. Two poultices a day will always draw out more pus than one, and remember to continue poulticing for 48 hours after all the discharge has apparently stopped. The hole must then be plugged (covered) to prevent further infection getting in. This can be done either under a shoe and a pad using a mixture of oakum and pine tar or tow and Stockholm Tar or filling wall defects with one of the modern synthetic horn replacers.

THRUSH

Thrush is an infection of the soft horn of the frog which occurs when the horse stands in damp conditions, e.g. when the bedding is not changed sufficiently often. It should be a rare condition because stable management should not allow the infection to gain a hold, but unfortunately it is still relatively common.

When a horse has thrush the frog itself, especially along the grooves where the frog joins the sole (page 57) and along the middle groove in the frog, becomes soft and infected with a damp, black, smelly pus. The resulting inflammatory reaction in the foot gives rise to heat and lameness. The first stage of treatment is to remove the predisposing damp conditions. Then the infected horn is cut away and a powerful antiseptic agent such as formalin is carefully applied daily to kill off any remaining infection.

The sole of the foot.

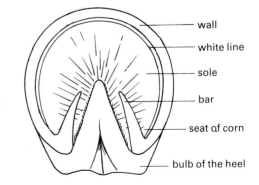

- wall
- white line
- sole
- bar
- seat of corn
- bulb of the heel

CORNS

A corn is a bruising of horn on the angle of the sole at the heel of the foot. This area is the so-called 'seat of corn'. One cause of the bruising is

Remedial shoes.

Anchor or 'T' shoe for treating corns combined with a contracted foot; all weight is taken by the frog.

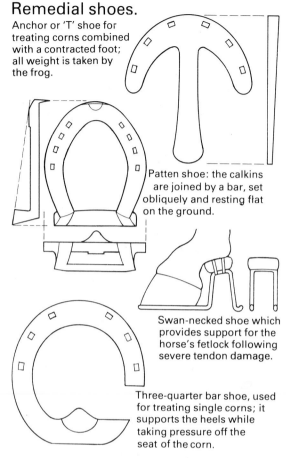

Patten shoe: the calkins are joined by a bar, set obliquely and resting flat on the ground.

Swan-necked shoe which provides support for the horse's fetlock following severe tendon damage.

Three-quarter bar shoe, used for treating single corns; it supports the heels while taking pressure off the seat of the corn.

basically that the shoe does not fit properly, and so presses on the sole rather than on the wall of the foot. Some horses, either by their action or because of the make-up of their feet, are extremely susceptible to corns and require constant attention to their feet.

When a horse is lame because of a corn, there is often nothing to see or feel until after the shoe has been removed. Even then it may take some paring down of the horn before the bruising is seen as a moist, red, discoloured area. Usually the discolouration is just blood from the bruising but sometimes infections can become established and black pus will be present. The pain is due to the presence of fluids from the blood where the horn cannot expand to make room for them. The treatment thus consists of cutting away all the bruised horn, and so removing the source of the pain. A special shoe should then be fitted which does not touch the hoof over the affected area, and thus lessens the percussion (concussion) on the site.

Diseases of tendons and muscles

THE ANATOMY OF THE LEG

Because we use our horses for movement it is not surprising that the means of movement, the legs, show so many signs of wear in the horse. It is important to realize that there are no muscles below the level of the knee or hock; the muscles which move the leg and foot are all situated some distance away from where they exert their effect.

Many people are confused with the terms 'tendons' and 'ligaments', but it is quite easy to distinguish which is which. A tendon is the fibrous 'rope' which transfers the pull exerted by a muscle from the muscle itself to the part of the body which has to be moved. A ligament is a

Tendons of the lower leg.

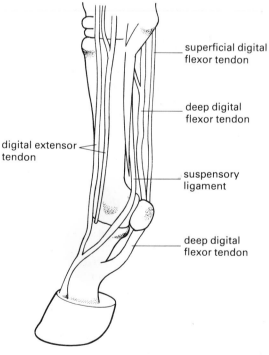

superficial digital flexor tendon

deep digital flexor tendon

digital extensor tendon

suspensory ligament

deep digital flexor tendon

band of tissue which holds two bones in position. When we talk about a horse's 'tendons' we almost always mean the tendons which run down the lower half of his leg and which are responsible for moving the foot.

The foot is pulled forward by the common digital extensor tendon, which runs all the way down the front of the leg to the foot itself. Because the leg is not under any strain when the leg is pulled forward, being off the ground at the time, this tendon does not have to be terribly strong.

The flexor tendons, on the other hand, which lie down the back of the leg, come under terrific strain because the leg is both bearing weight and moving when they are in use. There are two flexor tendons. The superficial flexor tendon is the most posterior, i.e. back one; it forms the rear outline of the leg. The superficial flexor tendon attaches around the horse's pastern. The deep flexor tendon lies just underneath the superficial flexor tendon, and the two tendons feel like one unit to the touch. The deep flexor tendon passes down over the navicular bone and attaches to the pedal bone. In order to help limit the amount of 'give' in this tendon there is another band of fibrous tissue, the check ligament, which extends down for a few cm/a couple of inches from behind the knee onto the tendon itself.

The bulge which you can feel on a horse's leg between the cannon bone and the flexor tendons is the suspensory ligament. This runs from just below the knee down to the fetlock joint, where it divides into two, each branch having a small pyramid-shaped accessory bone. These bones act as a kind of fulcrum or turning point, because the two branches of the suspensory ligament then go forward to attach on the lower front surface of the pastern.

Each tendon is made up of spindle-shaped bundles of collagen fibres. Most of these fibres run in the approximate direction of the greatest strain. The fibres have a small amount of elasticity, and in addition the bundles of fibres can move a little on one another. Mixed in with the collagen bundles are elastic fibres and blood vessels. Over the joints, each tendon runs inside a tendon sheath, with a lubricating fluid to ensure free movement up and down.

At the fetlock joint the tendons, and their tendon sheaths, pass through the capsule which surrounds the joint. This capsule extends a short way up the back of the leg above the joint. Wear and tear can cause this part of the capsule to become swollen with extra joint fluid, but this does not cause lameness at all. This condition is called 'windgalls' or 'windpuffs', and is only a blemish.

TENDON STRAIN AND ITS TREATMENT

When we consider that in a galloping horse 500–600 kg (1102–1323 lb) of weight is being supported by the very small cross-sectional area of the flexor tendons, it is hardly surprising that horses suffer from tendon problems. Different people have different definitions as to what constitutes a tendon sprain or strain. I propose to use the term 'tendon strain' for all injuries. Strains arise because of over-extension or over-stretching of the tendon. The pulling force is stronger than the natural elasticity of the tendon and the structure of the collagen fibres etc. is disrupted. Obviously a disrupted tendon loses some of its tensile strength, and so is more prone to further damage.

When a strain occurs there is always some damage to the blood vessels inside the tendon, and blood and tissue fluid are released into the tendon itself and the surrounding tissue. The structure of the bundles of fibres becomes disrupted, and the attachments between adjacent bundles are broken down. The tendon sheath (covering) is also affected. The sheath lining may become thickened or inflamed and release more fluid into the space between it and the actual tendon.

There are several common types of tendon injury which occur in riding horses.

Tenovitis

Tenovitis refers to an inflammation of the tendon sheath alone, which does not basically affect the tendon. The tendon area will be swollen and warm to the touch, and there may be a little oedema present. This oedema is tissue fluid which accumulates around the tendon sheath, and it can be easily recognised because when you press your fingers firmly into an area of oedema, they make pits which remain when

61

you remove your fingers (as against pressing into a collection of pus, where the indentations fill as soon as you remove your fingers). Often, though, the swelling is confined to the sheath itself which is swollen due to the presence of an increased amount of tendon fluid between the sheath and the tendon which it surrounds.

Bowed tendon on a right foreleg.

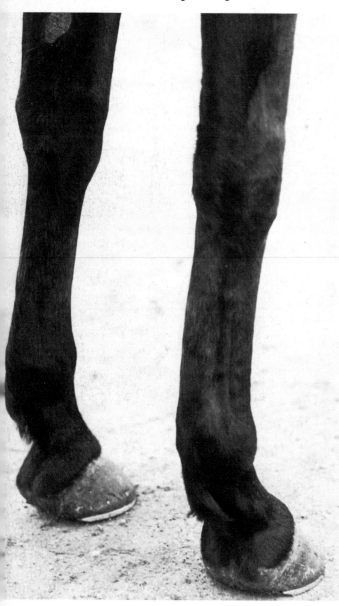

Common sites of tendon strains.

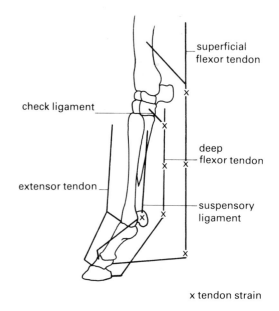

superficial flexor tendon

check ligament

deep flexor tendon

extensor tendon

suspensory ligament

x tendon strain

Bowed tendon

A horse's tendon may be said to be bowed. This is a warning sign. It is a serious warning, but it does not necessarily indicate serious trouble at the moment. The bowing is due to the release of blood and tissue fluid from slightly damaged blood vessels within the tendon. These small amounts of fluid thicken the tendon to the touch. If excessive strain is put on a bowed tendon, further and more serious damage will occur.

Strained tendon

When a tendon is strained the whole tendon area will become swollen with oedema. The area around the tendons will be warm to the touch and painful, and the horse will be markedly lame. The final stage is when the pulling forces have been so great that the tendon itself is ruptured. In addition to the above symptoms, the horse will no longer be supporting any weight on the tendon, even at rest. This means that if, for instance, the superficial flexor tendon is ruptured, the fetlock will sink down towards the ground.

The first and obvious treatment for tendon injuries is rest. Rest prevents further damage occurring and allows healing to take place. During the initial stages of the injury, when warmth over the site of the damage indicates that active inflammation is present, then rest means confinement to the loose box (box stall or small pen). When this active stage is over, possibly after about three weeks in the case of an actual tendon strain, then rest means confinement to a loose box (box stall) with one or two short periods of walking in-hand every day. These short periods of walking, which seem at odds with more traditional methods of treating tendon strains, ensure that gentle tension is placed on the new collagen fibres being formed and that these fibres are formed in the direction of pull and not haphazardly as would otherwise be the case. The result is a stronger repair. Rest does not mean turning the horse loose in a field, because a horse can gallop just as much loose in a field as it can with a rider on its back. Time spent in the field comes later in the period of convalescence for basically recovered tendons rather than part of the treatment.

Every owner of a horse with any degree of tendon damage always wants to know how long it will need to be rested. There are no set rules, your veterinary surgeon (veterinarian) will judge every case on its merits. A severe strain might need 9, 12, or up to 18 months rest before the healing is completed. One thing has now been proved conclusively, and that is that NO TREATMENT FOR TENDON INJURIES SPEEDS UP THE RECOVERY RATE. No matter what claims you might hear for this or that method of treatment, no particular treatment will result in your horse being ready for work any quicker. Some treatments will result in better and stronger healing, but none in any quicker healing.

The second basic treatment for tendon injuries is the application of cold. The cold causes contraction of the blood vessels in the inflamed area, and so less tissue fluid etc. accumulates. This is important because these fluids can 'clot' and form adhesions which will affect future movement. The pressure from fluid is the major cause of pain in the injured area. So keep the area as cold as you can by cold water bandaging, cold kaolin or other poultices, or one of those special dressings which you cool in the refrigerator and which then retain the cold when

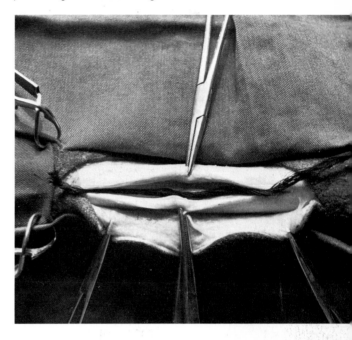

Carbon fibre operation: the carbon fibres are laid into place along a slit in the damaged tendon.

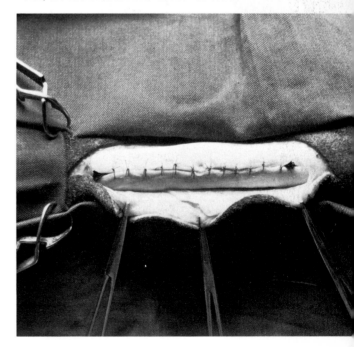

The tendon sheath is sutured over the rope of carbon fibres, the two ends of which can still be seen.

you place them on the horse's leg. Frequent changing of dressings will be necessary, as you will be amazed how quickly an inflamed leg heats up the dressing. A 'poultice boot' may be useful for keeping poultices in place.

The third basic treatment is the provision of support. Firm (but not tight) bandaging of both good and bad legs will help limit any further swelling around the tendons. It will also provide support to both the damaged tendons and those which are having to carry more weight because the horse is resting the affected leg.

The final basic treatment is the use of drugs to remove the oedema and to reduce the inflammation. A sudden tendon strain is an emergency. If you contact your veterinary surgeon (veterinarian) as soon as it happens and the horse goes lame, he will be able to help you to prevent the worst of the symptoms ever appearing. If, on the other hand, you wait several days until the inflammatory process is firmly established, treatment will have far less effect on the course of the healing process. In addition to the use of diuretics, such as frusemide, to reduce the oedema there are a whole host of anti-inflammatory drugs which are used. One factor which

your veterinary surgeon (veterinarian) will consider is whether it is desirable to use a drug with pain-killing effects or not. Most non-steroidal anti-inflammatory drugs do have a pain killing effect. If it is preferred not to mask the extent of healing in this way then a drug such as orgotein would have to be used instead. Orgotein is a non-steroidal anti-inflammatory drug which has no pain-killing effect.

In discussing the basic treatment of tendon injuries I have made no reference to either blistering (the application of an irritant substance to the skin over the tendons) or to firing (the insertion of red hot needles either into the depth of the tendon or partly through the overlying skin). This is because we now know that neither of these barbaric treatments has any value at all in speeding up healing of tendon strains. (Nor have drugs.) Hopefully the days are now over when these extremely painful 'treatments' were demanded routinely by horse owners.

There are two surgical techniques which I ought to mention. As I said earlier, these techniques do not result in the horse returning to the racetrack or hunting field any earlier, but

The muscles of the horse.

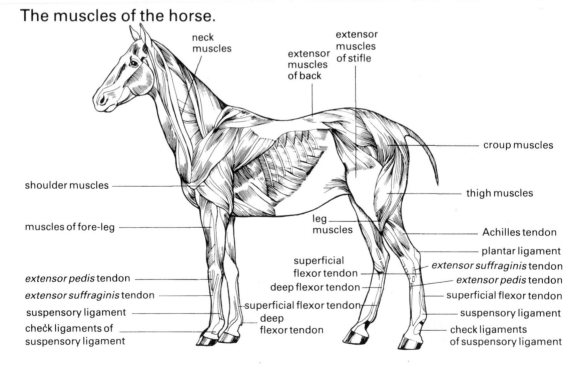

neck muscles

extensor muscles of back

extensor muscles of stifle

croup muscles

shoulder muscles

thigh muscles

muscles of fore-leg

leg muscles

Achilles tendon

plantar ligament

extensor pedis tendon

superficial flexor tendon

extensor suffraginis tendon

extensor suffraginis tendon

deep flexor tendon

extensor pedis tendon

suspensory ligament

superficial flexor tendon

superficial flexor tendon

suspensory ligament

deep flexor tendon

check ligaments of suspensory ligament

check ligaments of suspensory ligament

they may result in a more normal tendon after healing in severe cases. In a tendon splitting operation vertical cuts are made in the tendon at the affected area to allow blood vessels to penetrate from the surface into the centre of the tendon. These blood vessels should ensure more complete healing. More recently carbon fibres have been used in the repair of cut or ruptured tendons. A 'rope' of thousands of thin fibres of carbon is placed across, or in a vertical incision through the affected area of the tendon. The tendon is then sutured (stitched) around the fibres. In this case the carbon fibres do not take any strain. They act simply as a very efficient scaffolding along which the horse rapidly lays down new collagen fibres.

MUSCLE STRAINS

Muscle strains in the horse are comparatively uncommon. The muscles of movement are basically stronger and less prone to injury than the tendons through which they exert their pull. Of course, if a horse falls whilst jumping there will be damage to the muscles due to general bruising etc., but this heals readily.

The complex mass of muscles around the horse's shoulder can suffer from strain, usually as a result of injury whilst jumping. Anti-inflammatory drugs will relieve the pain involved but adequate rest is essential, otherwise the first time the horse jumps the muscle fibres will tear again on landing. It is perhaps not inappropriate to think of muscles as larger, softer tendons with a much greater blood supply, and muscle fibres which actually contract rather than the bundles of collagen fibres which merely resist stretching.

AZOTURIA (TIE-UP, SET-FAST, MONDAY MORNING DISEASE)

There is one major condition of the muscles which every horse owner should know about, understand and always take active measures to prevent, and that is azoturia or set-fast or tie-up. It is a management disease, and you are to blame if your horse succumbs to it. Because it is bad management which is responsible for causing azoturia, it is included here rather than in the chapter on feeding.

In the normal state of affairs you should aim to feed your horse just enough carbohydrate food, e.g. oats or pony nuts, grain or feed mix, to supply the energy which your horse will need during that particular day for whatever activity might be involved. If the horse consumes more carbohydrate than it needs, some of it is stored in the muscles of the body as an excess of a starch called glycogen. The muscles along the back and over the hindquarters are the main sites of glycogen storage. The beauty of glycogen as a future energy supply is that it can be 'burnt' and converted to energy without using any oxygen. So when the muscles are working hard but the oxygen supply from the blood stream is insufficient for their normal needs, they switch to glycogen. This releases energy, and results in the formation of lactic acid. This should be rapidly removed by the circulation, because if it is allowed to accumulate it will burn and destroy some of the muscle fibres.

Azoturia is a painful stiffness of the muscles of the hindquarters which is caused by muscle damage due to spasm of the blood vessels and accumulation of lactic acid. The stiffness always occurs during, or soon after, a period of exercise. There are several situations which predispose to this condition. If you feed a horse more carbohydrates than are necessary for the work he is doing, perhaps in your anxiety to have the horse in good condition for a particular event, then he can get azoturia. If you feed a horse for normal work but rest the horse for one or two days, then he can get azoturia (hence another name for the condition, Monday Morning Disease). If you feed a horse for normal work but then suddenly give him much more strenuous work, then he can get azoturia. Travelling long distances can prevent staling and lead to azoturia (tie-up) – especially in geldings who are reluctant to stale in this situation.

In all these cases the horse will become stiff and unwilling to move. He may even become recumbent and unable to rise. Because some muscle tissue is destroyed, there are various waste substances which are produced, and carried away via the blood stream which the horse attempts to remove through the kidneys into his urine. Unfortunately these molecules are often too large for the 'pores' in the filtering system within the kidneys. In the worst cases, the kidneys become blocked and the horse is unable to pass any urine. In less severe instances the urine is often dark red/brown in colour. The pain associated with azoturia can be so great that the horse may run a fever.

This, then, is the dramatic picture in an acute case of azoturia. Increasingly nowadays, veterinary surgeons (veterinarians) also see a sub-acute form. This is shown by the horse which is perfectly normal at rest in the stable but which sweats profusely whenever asked to trot or do fast work, failing to move freely. In this case the symptoms vanish as soon as the horse is returned to the stable.

Azoturia always involves physical damage to the muscles, no matter how slight. This results in the release of certain enzymes, notably creatine phosphokinase (C.P.K.), which are normally confined to within the muscle cells. The diagnosis of the disease can be readily confirmed by testing a blood sample for the levels of C.P.K. present. Raised blood levels of this substance only occur when muscle damage is present.

Treatment is obviously aimed at removing the symptoms. We have the complication, however, that any exercise before the condition is cured is liable to result in more lactic acid formation, more muscle damage and more symptoms. It is often, therefore, advisable to ask your veterinary surgeon (veterinarian) to carry out a check blood test before returning the horse to work. It may take weeks or even months of complete stable rest for the C.P.K. levels in the blood to return to normal, but the condition will not be cured until they do so.

If your horse exhibits symptoms of azoturia, stop work and rest him immediately, and keep him warmly wrapped up. The use of a potent diuretic which increases the kidney's ability to remove the dangerous waste products results in the horse passing urine again. Once the horse is able to carry out normal kidney function he will be in much less pain. Obviously anti-inflammatory drugs will counteract some of the destructive effects of the acid. It is claimed that naproxen is much more effective in the treatment of azoturia than other drugs such as cortisone or phenylbutazone. In Britain the use of naproxen is unfortunately limited by its very

high cost. Vitamin E and selenium preparations are also often given, in order to speed up the rate of muscle healing. These drugs are, however, no substitute for proper management (including restricting the horse's diet). This includes balancing the diet and exercise regime; and, in the high performance horse, the routine use of electrolyte drinks after hard exercise, and possibly the use of a supplement rich in vitamin E and selenium.

Diseases of the skeleton

BACK PROBLEMS
In recent years back problems have become more frequently diagnosed in horses. Various reasons have been advanced for this. Some people feel that the courses we expect our showjumpers and eventers to complete are too stiff and put too much strain on our horses. Other people point to the fact that self-styled chiropracters, who have no restrains on advertising and who never have to submit their results for analysis, have realized that there are many in the horse world ripe for exploitation. In the veterinary field, modern high-power radiography machines have certainly made diagnosis of some back problems easier, whilst surgical techniques have offered visible and dramatic means of treatment.

I must state here that horses do not actually displace vertebrae in their backs, whatever chiropracters may claim. If they did, the displaced bones would show on radiographs (which they never do). Indeed even in a dead horse, with no resistance to moving the vertebrae, displaced vertebrae are neither found nor can they be made to occur. Just under a half of all back injuries in the horse are due to soft tissue injuries, that is, they involve the muscles and ligaments of the back, with a similar proportion of cases involving the actual bony vertebrae.

Muscle strains usually occur during exercise, and affect all types and ages of horse. Often the pain causes a noticeable change of temperament in the horse, and the back is kept rigid. There is a ligament, the supraspinous ligament, which runs down the middle of the back and links the vertebrae. If this ligament is involved then recovery is much slower. Treatment of these injuries firstly involves rest. It makes sense not to aggravate an existing injury. Initially anti-inflammatory drugs will help to relieve the pain and remove the underlying inflammation. Niagara therapy, a cyclo-vibratory massage transmitted through a shaped cushion, is very effective in such cases, the massage effect reducing the fluid which is trapped so painfully in the damaged tissues. There are also other forms of physiotherapy equipment which in the hands of experts can help reduce inflammation. It is these cases also where chiropracters can achieve success. This is perhaps not because they have moved bones but because pressure at certain vital points removes the pain and so relaxes the muscle spasm which has built up (in effect, a form of acupuncture).

Back injuries can affect horses in ways which may not at first seem to be what one might

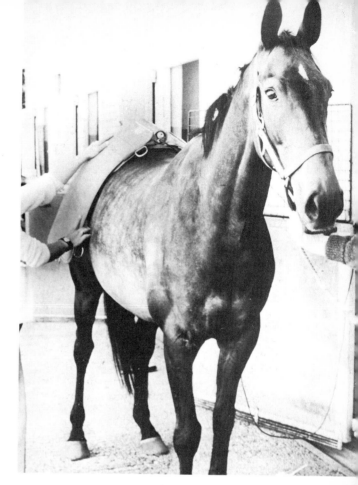

Using a special 'Equissage' Niagara pad in the treatment of a back injury; this is also used for loins, quarters and shoulders. Smaller hand units are used for a variety of injuries to other parts of the body.

The skeleton of the horse.

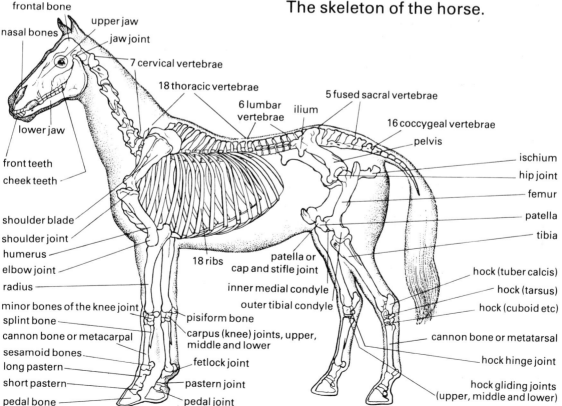

frontal bone
nasal bones
upper jaw
jaw joint
7 cervical vertebrae
18 thoracic vertebrae
6 lumbar vertebrae
ilium
5 fused sacral vertebrae
16 coccygeal vertebrae
pelvis
ischium
hip joint
femur
patella
tibia
lower jaw
front teeth
cheek teeth
shoulder blade
shoulder joint
humerus
elbow joint
radius
18 ribs
patella or cap and stifle joint
inner medial condyle
outer tibial condyle
minor bones of the knee joint
splint bone
cannon bone or metacarpal
sesamoid bones
long pastern
short pastern
pedal bone
pisiform bone
carpus (knee) joints, upper, middle and lower
fetlock joint
pastern joint
pedal joint
hock (tuber calcis)
hock (tarsus)
hock (cuboid etc)
cannon bone or metatarsal
hock hinge joint
hock gliding joints (upper, middle and lower)

expect. Chronic strain of the sacro-illiac ligament, which joins the pelvis to the spine, often
does not affect the horse's ability to jump but the
horse may be in obvious pain when only
trotting. This is because the horse can use the
back muscles as a 'splint' at fast paces, but
cannot do so during more flexible activities.

The most common condition affecting the
bones of the back is crowding and over-riding of

Over-riding of the dorsal spinous processes.

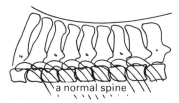

a normal spine

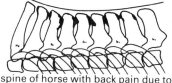

areas of new bone formed where adjacent
processes rub against one another

spine of horse with back pain due to
over-riding of the dorsal processes

the dorsal spinous processes. This occurs especially at that part of the back, just at the rear of
the saddle area, where the dorsal processes of the
vertebrae change their direction. There is an
inbuilt tendency for crowding in this region.
Radiographic confirmation of such bony back
problems can only be carried out at a few
specialist centres due to the extremely powerful
radiography machines necessary. Veterinary
surgeons (veterinarians) can, however, use infil-
trations of local anaesthetic to show that bony,
rather than muscle, changes are at the root of the
problem. In some of these cases, radical surgery
to remove the arthritic bone has been very
successful in enabling affected horses to return
to normal work. The cost of such a large scale
operation is, of course, very high and it is worth
noting that at least one critical survey reports
that rest alone is just as effective as surgery in
curing this condition in many horses.

SPLINTS

Although few horses will suffer major back
problems during their lifetime, many (possibly
the majority of horses) will develop one or more
splints. A splint is a lump of new bone which
forms at the junction of one of the splint bones
and the cannon bone. The scientific term for
such new bone formation is an exostosis.

What happens is that concussive forces travelling up the leg damage the ligament joining the
splint bone to the cannon bone and the new bone
is formed bridging the gap between these two
bones.

Splints occur most commonly on the fore legs,
which receive more percussion (concussion in
USA) during roadwork etc. than the hind legs.
They are also usually on the medial or inside
surface of the cannon. Many people look on
splints as occurring solely in young horses.
Although it is true that the softer bones of young
horses cannot withstand the pressures of work as
well as those of older horses, and splints are
often the result, they can occur in any age of
horse if circumstances put more percussion
(concussion) on a leg than the bone can stand.

Splints can appear without causing any pain
or lameness. Equally the inflamed bone surfaces
may cause pain and lameness for several weeks

Splint formation.

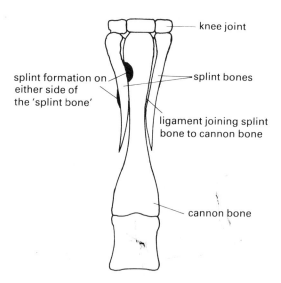

knee joint

splint formation on
either side of
the 'splint bone'

splint bones

ligament joining splint
bone to cannon bone

cannon bone

before actual new bone is formed. Usually the first sign is a warm swelling along the junction of the bones. If the horse becomes lame, this lameness increases with exercise, especially with trotting or jumping on hard surfaces (which can even include grass fields during the summer time). Rest and frequent cold applications, e.g. cold water bandages or cold kaolin, are usually all that are required in the way of treatment. The inflamed bone settles down, the normal covering membrane grows over it, and the horse becomes sound again.

In more severe cases, or in cases where, for one reason or another, the horse has continued to work despite developing splint problems, veterinary treatment may be necessary. Giving pain-killing drugs by mouth or by injection is not very successful in such cases, and local treatments are used. Cortisone, either 'painted' onto the area or injected around the splint, is a common treatment. As always when using such drugs, it is important not to work the horse too soon; the horse may well be free of pain before he is free of inflammation. In extreme cases, where your veterinary surgeon (veterinarian) is sure that no fractures etc. are present but where the splint remains painful, surgery or firing may be employed.

SPAVIN

A spavin is a bony enlargement on the inside of the hock due to an osteoarthritis between adjacent bones in the hock. It arises due to stress, and is especially common in young horses with narrow tapering hocks. Initially there is a lameness which wears off with exercise, and then the new bone formation becomes visible. Because the horse can no longer bend the hock joint as freely as before, the toe tends to be dragged rather than lifted clear of the ground. Painful tension when the hock is fully extended causes the horse to snatch the leg up at each stride. Even at rest the foot may be pointed, or rested, in order to rest the hock. As the condition progresses, the horse becomes permanently lame.

There is a simple 'spavin test' for determining whether a horse has a spavin. This consists of forcibly flexing the hock, and holding it bent for about thirty seconds before releasing the leg and trotting the horse straight away. Unfortunately painful lesions elsewhere in the leg will also cause increased lameness following the spavin test. Where there is any doubt, local nerve blocks or radiographs will confirm the diagnosis.

Treatment of a spavin relies on encouraging fusion of the two bones, as it is movement of these arthritic bones which causes the pain. This fusion may occur naturally following sufficient rest. It may be speeded up by alternating rest with periods of exercise and non-steroid anti-inflammatory drugs. When this does not happen, surgical fusion may well be necessary.

There is another condition of the hock with the confusing name of 'bog spavin'. This is a swelling of the joint capsules around the hock which occurs on the medial surface of the joint. It is commonly seen in horses with upright hocks. The swelling is not painful and does not cause lameness. Pressure bandaging and cold compresses may decrease the swelling but will not usually remove it completely.

An X-ray of a bone spavin.

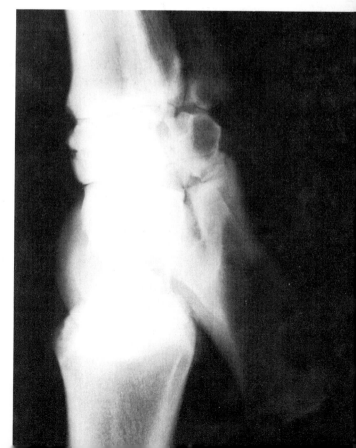

The site of spavin in the hock.

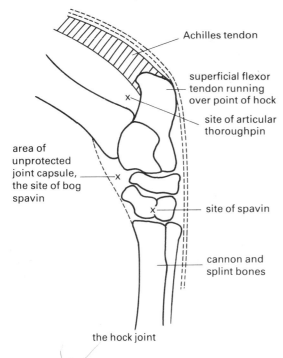

Achilles tendon

superficial flexor tendon running over point of hock

site of articular thoroughpin

area of unprotected joint capsule, the site of bog spavin

site of spavin

cannon and splint bones

the hock joint

CURBS

A curb is a swelling directly on the back of the hock due to a sprain of the plantar ligament which joins the cannon bone to the bottom row of bones in the hock. As with most sprains, swelling and lameness develop. Often this condition is the result of pulling a horse up sharply on its haunches or of over extension of the hock during jumping. Horses with sickle shaped hocks are thought to be more susceptible to curbs than horses with better conformation.

Initially the standard trio of anti-inflammatory treatments should be used (rest, cold and anti-inflammatory drugs). Even though the lameness may disappear, the swelling will remain. Horses which have sprained the plantar ligament once are always liable to do so again when the joint is under great strain.

RINGBONE

Ringbone in the horse is the classic form of arthritis. If it affects the pastern joint it is known as high ringbone; if it affects the joint between the pedal (coffin) bone and the pastern, it is

known as low ringbone. New bone is formed all around the joint (hence the name 'ringbone'), and there is progressive lameness. Pain-killing drugs such as phenylbutazone may enable the horse to return to work, but failing this, surgical cutting of the nerves (neurectomy) may be the only hope of removing the pain associated with this condition.

OTHER BONE CONDITIONS

Young horses have 'softer' bone which is less able to withstand the stresses of work than the bone of mature horses. Young Thoroughbreds in training, for example, often develop sore shins, when the bone is painful but not necessarily physically changed. The growth centres in the immature bones are also vulnerable. Epiphysitis is an inflammation of a growth plate, causing swelling, heat and pain. With rest these conditions resolve themselves, although epiphysitis may leave some swelling of the joint.

Sometimes even mature bone can develop hair-line 'stress cracks', with resulting lameness. Complete rest will allow healing to occur.

Not all bony changes necessarily cause lameness. Pedal ostitis is a condition where areas of the pedal bone become less dense. Many older horses show these changes on radiographic examination, but not all these horses show any signs of lameness. When lameness does occur, treatment is with anti-inflammatory drugs, usually phenylbutazone.

FINAL THOUGHTS ON LAMENESS

There are three points which have been mentioned time and time again in this chapter.

1 The need for accurate early diagnosis.
2 Rest is the first stage of any treatment for diseases of movement.
3 Anti-inflammatory drugs work best during the early stages of a condition, when active inflammation is present, so if veterinary treatment is to achieve maximum effectiveness it must start as early as possible.

Please remember these points even if you forget all the detail of the specific causes of lameness.

7 Diseases of breeding

The normal pregnancy

A normal pregnancy starts with a normal oestrus cycle, or 'heat', so we must understand what this term 'oestrus' means. It has been defined as 'the recurrent restricted period of sexual receptivity during which changes are produced in the genital organs as a result of hormonal activity'. The cycle has a period lasting about 16 days when the mare shows no sexual interest at all, due to the presence in her ovaries of a small piece of tissue called a corpus luteum which secretes the hormone progesterone. As this corpus luteum starts to die away, one or more follicles develop in one of the ovaries. These follicles are small, fluid-filled sacs which have an egg inside them. At this stage more hormonal changes cause the mare to become sexually

The reproductive tract.

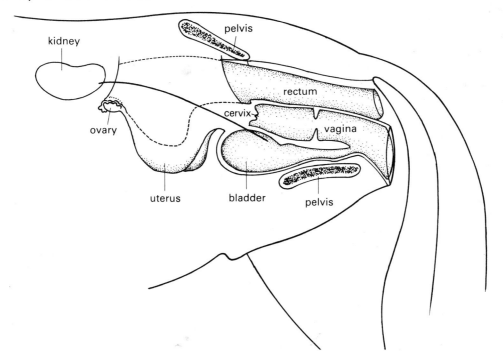

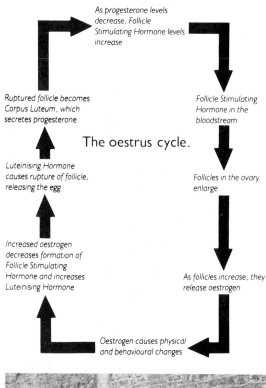

The oestrus cycle.

As progesterone levels decrease, Follicle Stimulating Hormone levels increase

Ruptured follicle becomes Corpus Luteum, which secretes progesterone

Follicle Stimulating Hormone in the bloodstream

Luteinising Hormone causes rupture of follicle, releasing the egg

Follicles in the ovary enlarge

Increased oestrogen decreases formation of Follicle Stimulating Hormone and increases Luteinising Hormone

As follicles increase, they release oestrogen

Oestrogen causes physical and behavioural changes

receptive. This period of oestrus culminates in ovulation, when the follicle ruptures and releases the ripe egg.

If the mare is not mated (bred), then the ruptured follicle becomes a corpus luteum, and the cycle is turning again. If the mare is mated by a stallion within about 48 hours before ovulation, one of the stallion's sperm (and around 15,000 million sperm are ejaculated into the mare at each mating) will almost certainly meet up with the fertile egg inside the mare and fertilization will occur. The mare must now stop the cycle because if another oestrus period occurs, the uterine environment will become quite unsuitable for the fertilized egg, which will die. The corpus luteum in such 'pregnant' mares persists and prevents any more oestrus cycles. During the first month of pregnancy small follicles appear in the ovaries which change into secondary corpora lutea in order to provide further progesterone to keep the cycling activity

Stallion nuzzling mare over the teasing board. Note that the mare, who is in season, is accepting his attentions quietly.

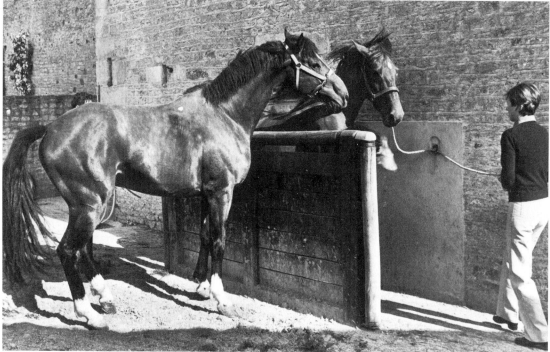

dampened down. The mare's pregnancy usually lasts on average 340 days, but its length is so variable that a pregnancy lasting anywhere between 320 and 360, even 370 days is considered perfectly normal.

DETECTION OF OESTRUS, OR HEAT

In the natural state the stallion decides when the mare is in oestrus and ready for mating. He does this a lot more efficiently than man ever manages to do. Obviously the mare shows she is in oestrus by becoming willing to accept mating with the stallion, rather than attempting to kick him away as she would during the rest of her cycle. Stud farms may 'tease' the mare by bringing a stallion close in order to watch her reaction, without actually allowing mating to take place, often using a teasing board.

Mares 'in heat' or in oestrus often squat slightly and hold their tail to one side as if to expose the vulva. The vulva 'winks' open and shut, often releasing small quantities of urine. Another sign of oestrus is clear mucus draining from the vulva.

PREVENTION OF SEXUALLY TRANSMITTED INFECTIONS

There are some infections of the mare's genital tract which can infect the stallion at mating and then be passed on to further mares when he mates them. As the presence of infections invariably results in infertility, these infections are very serious when they occur. As recently as 1977 an entirely new infection appeared in the Thoroughbred population of Western Europe, Contagious Equine Metritis (C.E.M.). Despite vigorous measures to control this and other sexually transmitted infections, outbreaks still occur.

Prevention of these diseases is based on swabbing various areas of the mare's genital tract and then culturing the swabs in an incubator in the laboratory to see whether any infectious organism grows or not. An infected mare must be treated and not served (bred). When a mare's cervix or uterine wall is swabbed, this must be carried out during oestrus if reliable results are to be obtained. This method is often used to detect Pseudomonas, Klebsiella and C.E.M. infections, and will also detect ordinary

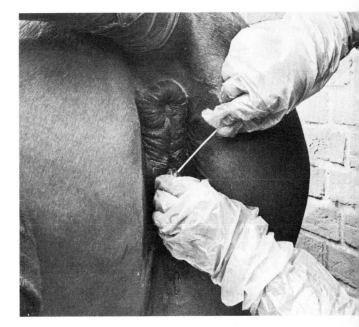

Veterinary surgeon (veterinarian) (wearing sterile gloves) taking a clitoral swab from a mare.

infections of the genital tract which might not be sexually transmitted. C.E.M. also manages to survive for very long periods in the clitoral sinuses just inside the mare's vulva. Swabbing to detect this organism may require repeated clitoral swabs, which may be taken at any stage of the oestrus cycle.

In the USA, the Coggins test will be necessary for any horses travelling between one state and another.

DETECTION OF PREGNANCY

Following an apparently successful mating, the mare owner wants to know as soon as possible whether the mare is pregnant or not. The mere fact that the mare is not observed to be in oestrus again is an indication, but not a very reliable one, that she is pregnant.

As early as 16 to 17 days after ovulation it is possible to take a blood sample and test this for levels of progesterone. If the mare is still cycling (and so not pregnant) the levels of this hormone should be almost zero at this time. High progesterone levels will indicate a possible pregnancy.

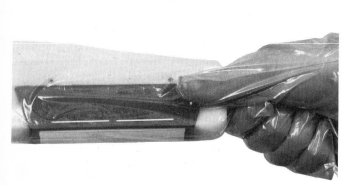

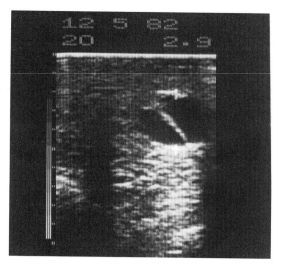

The use of echography for horses is almost exclusively for the detection of pregnancy. The ultra-sound probe *left* builds up a picture of the uterus *right*.

Manual examinations of the mare's uterus are carried out by veterinary surgeons (veterinarians), who insert an arm into the mare's rectum and feel the uterus through the rectal wall. This examination is usually undertaken at 42 days or later, although specialists may be able to detect the swelling in one of the uterine horns which indicates a pregnancy earlier than this.

There are also laboratory methods of detecting pregnancy. A blood sample taken between 40 and 110 days of pregnancy can be tested for levels in the blood of the hormone, progesterone. This test has the advantage of not disturbing the genital tract at all. After about 100 days of pregnancy the reliability of the blood test decreases, and during the second part of pregnancy confirmation is from a urine test for the hormone oestrogen.

The most recent development in pregnancy detection is the use of echography. Using an ultra-sound probe a cross-sectional picture of the uterus is built up. Although the equipment is extremely expensive at present, this appears to be the most reliable method of pregnancy detection developed so far. In the Thoroughbred and purebred field, where large sums of money are involved, this method will undoubtedly be widely used in the future.

ABORTION

One of the more frustrating aspects of horse breeding is the fact that so many properly fertilized eggs fail to result in a live foal eleven months later. It is sometimes thought that during the first six or seven weeks of pregnancy the embryo may be resorbed by the mare; this means that the embryo dies and is absorbed in situ, rather than expelled out of the uterus. This is one of the main reasons why a mare diagnosed in foal at 42 days of pregnancy fails to produce a foal. Even up to 100 days of pregnancy abortion is relatively common in the mare. At this stage the embryo is very small, and its expulsion may pass completely unnoticed. It has been suggested that this is due to lack of progesterone during pregnancy, and many mares are given progesterone implants to maintain their pregnancies. Usually the doses of hormone given are too low to exert any significant effect, but measurement of blood progesterone levels can both confirm the diagnosis and provide a guide as to proper treatment levels.

SEASONAL BREEDING ACTIVITY

Although human beings will conceive and give birth at any time of the year, horses are seasonal breeders. Mares only come into oestrus during the spring and summer, foaling at the same time in the following year when climate and food sources are favourable. Ponies usually do not cycle at all during the winter months, although

Thoroughbreds may cycle irregularly even during the winter period.

In the northern hemisphere the official Thoroughbred breeding season is February 15th to July 15th. In the southern hemisphere it runs from August 12th to January 15th. This is really too early, with the result that many mares will not naturally cycle in the early stages of the season. Artificial lights and warmth are often used to 'cheat' the mare into thinking that spring has arrived. It is also possible to feed the mare an orally active progesterone compound for a couple of weeks. When this is stopped the mare's hormonal system rebounds the other way, and the mare comes into oestrus.

Even during the natural breeding season a mare may fail to cycle for some reason (always remembering that the commonest reason for failing to cycle is pregnancy!). As long as the ovaries are not completely inactive, prostaglandin injections will often result in a mare coming into normal fertile oestrus about 4 to 6 days later.

Foaling

It is customary to divide the process of giving birth, or parturition, into three stages. These three stages of labour follow a regular pattern, but the problem in the horse is to know when to expect the first stage to begin. As I have already mentioned, pregnancies in the mare are very variable in their length. If northern hemisphere mares are mated in the December to April period, they tend to have a longer pregnancy than mares mated during the summer months. Colt foals also tend to be carried longer than filly foals.

You must therefore make your preparations for foaling in plenty of time. The first decision is whether you will allow the mare to foal outside or keep her inside. In some parts of the world, such as Australia and New Zealand, even the most expensive Thoroughbred mare may well be foaled outside. Under European conditions I personally advise that you plan to foal your mare inside as long as an adequate, clean stable is available. If the choice is between an unsatisfactory stable or foaling outside, on the other hand, I would choose to foal her outside.

Leaving your mare outside makes it more difficult to find her and check that all is well at night time when you suspect that foaling may be imminent. If something does go wrong, it is obviously easier to restrain the mare, and help her, inside a stable. The new-born foal will also find it easier to suckle the mare and form a good mare-foal bond in the more confined space.

Apart from a new 5 cm/2 in width cotton bandage, and some antibiotic spray, for use on the foal's navel, the most important preparation is to have your veterinary surgeon's (veterinarian's) telephone number instantly available. As will become obvious, most mares foal without any problems, but when difficulties do arise every minute can be important.

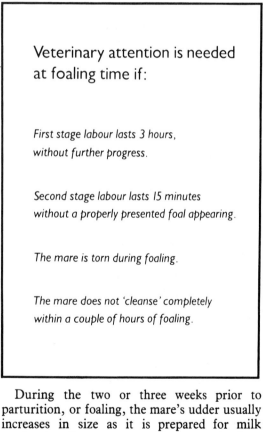

Veterinary attention is needed at foaling time if:

First stage labour lasts 3 hours, without further progress.

Second stage labour lasts 15 minutes without a properly presented foal appearing.

The mare is torn during foaling.

The mare does not 'cleanse' completely within a couple of hours of foaling.

During the two or three weeks prior to parturition, or foaling, the mare's udder usually increases in size as it is prepared for milk production. In some mares this preparation is so great that milk will stream from the udder for days before foaling. The first milk produced is very rich in antibodies against infection, and if this colostrum, as it is called, is lost, the foal will have no protection against infection during his first couple of months of life. If a mare does run with milk it is a good idea to milk about 1 litre (2 pints in USA/1¾ pints in Britain) of the colostrum into a sterilized container and store it in a deep freeze until the foal is born. It can be thawed and given to the foal during the first 8 hours of his life. The majority of mares develop a drop of honey-like secretion at the tip of their teats about 48 hours prior to foaling, which gives some warning that it is imminent.

STAGE ONE OF LABOUR

During the late stages of pregnancy the foal lies on his back inside the mare's uterus.

The foal in the mare's uterus, twisting round for delivery.

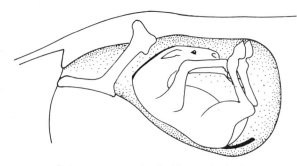

Late pregnancy: the foal lies on its back

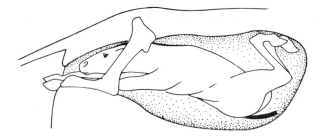

Early in parturition: the head and forelegs twist round into a diving position

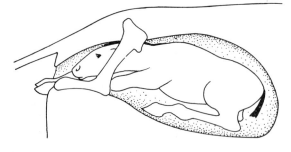

The actual birth: the head and forelegs pull the rest of the body round

During the early stages of parturition, or delivery, however, the foal starts to twist round for delivery. The first stage of labour almost always starts at night, even if the foaling box or area is lit artificially 24 hours of the day. It lasts about an hour, and ends when the first water bag bursts, releasing its fluid.

During this stage the mare becomes restless and may have colic-type pains in her abdomen. She often turns to look at her flanks, and patchy sweating may be visible. It may be possible to see foal movements showing through her abdominal wall.

There is not an awful lot to go wrong with the first stage of labour, although some mares may have 'false alarm' colics during the weeks before the actual birth. Occasionally the mare's uterine muscles may fail to start contracting. This inertia means that the mare is incapable of pushing the foal out of the uterus. If you think that the first stage of labour has gone on for 3 hours and still the mare has not started straining to push the foal out, call your veterinary surgeon (veterinarian).

STAGE TWO OF LABOUR

This is the stage of actual delivery. The uterine muscles contract forcefully, and the mare lies down. By now the foal has twisted round, so that he lies the right way up.

Forceful straining of the muscles of the mare's abdomen results in the appearance of a membranous sac at her vulva. Within an astonishingly short time, about 12 minutes, the foal has been pushed out inside this membrane, which is called the amnion. The foal's leg and neck movements usually break the amnion; if it fails to do so, assistance must be given. As the head is exposed, breathing begins. Delivery of the hind legs presents few problems; either the foal 'crawls' away or the mare's movements leave him behind.

Very strong forces must obviously be involved if such a large, long-legged offspring as a foal is to be delivered within minutes. The advantage of this is that with such powerful contractions the mare will usually manage to foal on her own if it is at all 'equinely' possible. The great disadvantage is that if the foal is not lying quite right inside the uterus then serious problems

arise. For example, if one of the foal's legs is bent backwards, the foal will become wedged into the mare's birth canal rather like a cork in a bottle. Alternatively the wrongly-positioned foal may be delivered but may damage the mare in the process.

It is important, therefore, to realise that any abnormality during the second stage of labour is an emergency. Do not delay, even for minutes. If, after a few minutes' effort, two feet and a muzzle do not appear, contact your veterinary surgeon (veterinarian) immediately. It is better to shout for help unnecessarily than to risk either a dead foal or a damaged mare (and possibly both). If the mare's vulva is torn at foaling, it will be necessary to perform a minor operation, called a Caslick's operation, to restore things to normal. This operation results in the vulval opening being reduced, and so the operation may need to be undone and resutured at both covering (breeding) and foaling times in the future.

Inside the uterus the foal is attached to and nurtured from the mare's own blood circulation through his umbilical cord. Even immediately after he has been born, this link will remain. It is very important that you do not sever this cord. Even after birth blood from the placenta (the layers of membranes which surround the foal inside the uterus) passes along the cord into the foal. If you sever the cord, you may deprive the foal of vital blood. The cord breaks naturally as the foal moves. If the stump left hanging from the foal continues to bleed, you should tie it off with a clean bandage or a length of catgut, dental floss, or similar etc. The cord stump should be dipped, sprayed or dusted with an antibiotic (antiseptic in USA) in order to prevent a navel infection becoming established.

STAGE THREE OF LABOUR

By this stage, we are no longer concerned with the foal. It is the cleaning out stage when the placental membranes are expelled from the mare's uterus. Normally this process takes about an hour. The placenta becomes inverted, so that when you see it, it is inside out. It is important that you do see the placenta, because you must check that it is complete. If any fragment is left behind inside the uterus it will quite rapidly

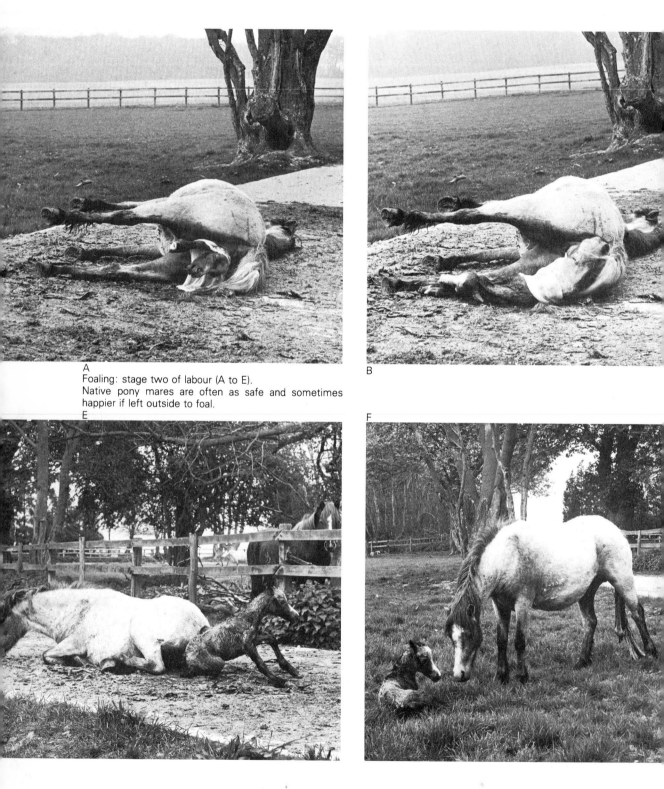

A

B

Foaling: stage two of labour (A to E).
Native pony mares are often as safe and sometimes happier if left outside to foal.

E

F

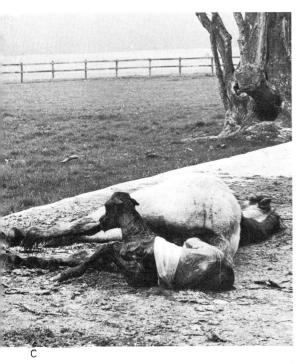

C

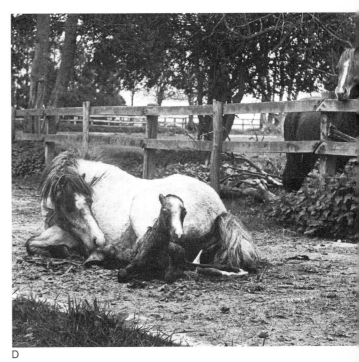

D

Foaling: stage three of labour (F to H) is completed and the Y-shaped afterbirth has been passed.

The foal finds its dam's udder.

G

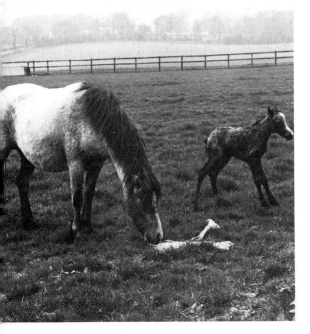

H

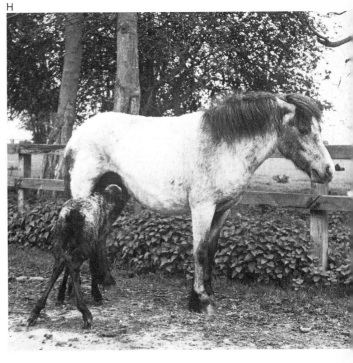

decompose and become infected. If the mare does not 'cleanse' properly, contact your veterinary surgeon (veterinarian). Even with modern antibiotics, this is a serious condition which could kill the mare if not treated properly. It can also cause laminitis.

Diseases of the foal

RETAINED MECONIUM
When a foal is born, his large colon already contains faeces. This represents some waste products of the foal's body functions in utero (i.e. before birth). This faecal material is called meconium, and it must be expelled from the body during the first few hours of life. Although both colts and fillies can retain their meconium, the anatomy of colts means 'hat they are far, far more likely to suffer from this condition than fillies.

A healthy foal will pass his meconium within 2 or 3 hours of birth. You can distinguish meconium from the normal faeces which will follow it by the colour. Meconium tends to be orangey yellow in colour rather than greeny brown. The appearance after it of normal-coloured faeces is a sign that all the meconium has been passed. Retention of these waste products rapidly leads to toxicity and colic. One of the first symptoms of retained meconium is that the foal either fails to suck at all, or starts to suck normally and then stops doing so. The foal may run a fever, and is listless. Initially he will strain frequently in an attempt to push out the meconium, which becomes more dry, and so more difficult to expel, with every hour.

You should not see the worst symptoms of retained meconium, because your observation of the foal should have led you to seek veterinary advice before any serious symptoms occur. Certainly you should watch the foal carefully until all the meconium has been expelled and normal faeces are being passed. It is not enough to just see a foal pass 4–5 cm/1½–2 in, or a handful of meconium, it must all come out. A foal is a delicate animal; if you allow a disease to progress to the stage where he stops suckling his mother's milk, you may have great trouble in getting him suckling again.

I would suggest that inexperienced people do not attempt to physically remove any meconium which is retained. Your veterinary surgeon (veterinarian) will probably use a combination of enemas and physical methods to achieve this aim. This is a potentially fatal ailment, so take no risks.

HAEMOLYTIC ANAEMIA
Although I have stressed the importance of ensuring that a foal receives his mother's colostrum during his first 12 hours of life, there is one rare situation where this brings problems as well as benefits. During pregnancy some of the foal's blood may leak back into the mare's bloodstream. If the mare's body considers this blood of an incompatible type, a foreign substance, antibodies will be produced against it. The colostrum will contain these antibodies just as it contains protective antibodies against various infections etc. When the foal drinks the colostrum these antibodies will attack his red blood cells. Because it destroys, or haemolyses, these blood cells, the resulting condition is called haemolytic anaemia.

The symptoms of haemolytic anaemia usually become apparent before the second or third day of the foal's life. The foal may be seen to breathe faster than normal, and its heart-beat or pulse can be felt to be faster also. The broken-down haemoglobin from the red blood cells causes severe jaundice, the membranes around his eyes and mouth becoming yellow in colour. The urine is tinged red with blood. Naturally the foal becomes dull and listless.

Veterinary attention is essential if you suspect this condition, but even whilst waiting for the veterinary surgeon (veterinarian) to arrive you should stop the foal suckling his mother. Treatment may necessitate giving the foal a blood transfusion. Once a mare has produced one haemolytic foal, there is a strong likelihood of her producing another one at subsequent foalings. It is possible to check the chance of this occurring by blood typing both the mare and the stallion to determine whether the resultant foal's blood is likely to stimulate the mare's body in this way or not. If you suspect a foal might be at risk, he should be prevented from suckling his own mother for the first 24 to 36 hours of life.

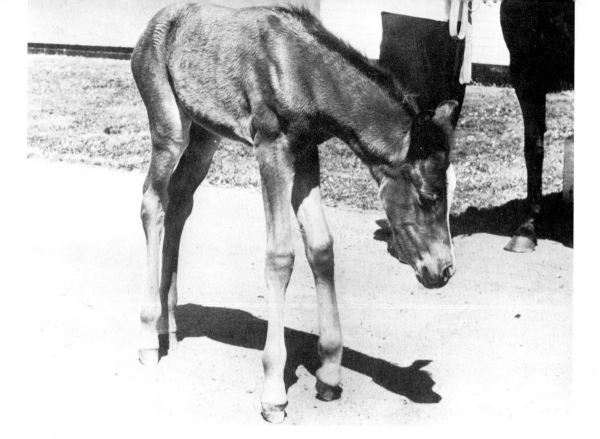

During this time the mare's milk should be milked out to remove the colostrum. The foal should be given the colostrum from another mare, and possibly fed an artificial milk substitute until it is safe to allow him to suckle his mother.

SCOURING

Diarrhoea in foals, as in any young animal, is potentially serious. It is not the cause of the diarrhoea which presents such problems, it is the foal's inability to compensate for the loss of so much fluid (containing as it does vital salts, etc.). It is normal for most foals to scour temporarily around nine or ten days after foaling, at the time their mother comes into oestrus for the so-called 'foaling heat'. This is because a mare in oestrus secretes substances into her milk which tend to cause diarrhoea in the foal. No treatment is usually necessary because the condition is not severe enough to cause serious fluid loss.

Various infections can also cause diarrhoea, and these are potentially more serious. The foal may run a fever and become weak and dehydrated. The fact that such a foal ceases to suckle

Foal with contracted flexor tendons. Note how upright the pastern bones are.

only makes the effects of dehydration worse. Treatment with antibiotics of any bacteria involved is important, but replacement of the lost salts and fluid (either orally or by injections etc.) is the measure which will save the foal's life.

We have to remember that even in the best managed stud or stable, a foal lives in a dirty environment, where bacteria such as Escherichia coli are present all the time. In addition to causing scouring, such bacteria may localise at the umbilicus (navel) and cause an infection of the umbilical cord (called 'navel ill'). Once they have gained access to the foal's bloodstream, bacteria may become lodged in the joints. The resulting 'joint ill' causes the affected joint to become hot and swollen. The damage to the joint surfaces etc. may become permanent and interfere with the animal's future use.

In order to prevent these infections in young foals some veterinary surgeons (veterinarians) recommend routine antibiotic injections during the first ten days of the foal's life. Although tetanus antitoxin can be given to even very young foals, vaccination against diseases such as tetanus or influenza cannot be started until the foal is at least three months old. This is because not until then is the foal's immune system mature enough to respond to vaccines *(page 11)*.

PHYSICAL ABNORMALITIES

You should always examine a new born foal for any physical abnormalities such as having an eye missing etc. At this stage you would also pick up umbilical hernias which may need treatment later. This is where a hole in the abdominal muscles allows some of the abdominal contents to escape and lie under the skin as a soft swelling. Occasionally foals are born with their flexor tendons apparently contracted. Support bandaging will often allow these foals to stand on the deformed limbs, and their own body weight gradually 'stretches' the tendons until they return to normal. A similar condition may arise later in life. If foals are fed too much on park-type pastures, it is thought by some veterinary surgeons in Britain that the bones may grow faster than the tendons do. Treatment consists of allowing the foal to lose weight until a balance is reached between the growth rates of the various structures in the legs. In the USA it is held that the growth plates in the legs become painful and lead to flexor muscle spasm and contractions, there being no evidence of differential growth. Treatment consists of feeding the foal so that it grows more slowly. It must be ensured that the whole diet is correctly balanced in terms of vitamins, minerals and amino acids.

Castration

Although castration is an operation carried out by choice, rather than an ailment, I think it merits a few words of explanation. Castration is the surgical removal of both testicles from a male horse, in order to remove the unwanted aspects of male behaviour. Even as an unweaned foal some males may pester their mother, attempting to mount her and risking injury to both parties. Some foals are thus castrated prior to or at weaning. More usually, horses not likely to be used for breeding are castrated at one year old.

At this age they have developed physically and mentally but are still reasonably easy to handle. Castrating older horses is perfectly possible, but an adult stallion can present handling difficulties. It is the unpredictable, domineering nature of stallions, especially in the presence of other horses, which makes castration such a common procedure.

In centuries past stallions were castrated in the standing position, whilst still conscious. Almost all modern veterinary surgeons in Britain now anaesthetise the animal and operate on the recumbent horse. Not only is this safer for the surgeon, it guarantees that he can operate by sight, not touch, and so be sure to remove all the necessary tissue.

RIGS (CRYPTORCHIDS, 'RIDGELINGS' IN USA)

In a small proportion of male horses, only one testicle descends fully into the scrotum (as the pouch of skin underneath the body for the testicles is called). These horses are known as rigs or cryptorchids. If this is the case, it is important never to operate and just remove the obvious testicle. If this is done, the hidden testicle is still capable of producing male hormone and so causing the undesirable features of male behaviour. Removing the one testicle does not speed up the descent of the other testicle.

If a horse appears to be a rig (cryptorchid), the veterinary surgeon (veterinarian) will sedate him and then examine him quietly at rest. The resulting relaxation often allows a testicle which is merely being held high up in its 'canal' to descend sufficiently for it to be felt. In these cases the hidden testicle is outside the abdominal cavity, and a comparatively straightforward form of ordinary castration will enable both testicles to be removed. If, however, the second testicle is still inside the abdomen, a major abdominal operation is necessary to remove it.

There are some castrated male horses which behave as though they are still stallions, much to the annoyance of their owners. Blood tests for possible male hormone will indicate whether a testicles or testicular tissue still remains, but in many of these cases the undesirable behaviour has no detectable cause.

8 Diseases of the skin

Skin infections

There are several general comments which apply to all skin infections of the horse. The first is that possession of a thick coat of hair tends to encourage such problems, because the handler often fails to diagnose that a problem exists until the condition is well established. Secondly, infected horses which are being groomed will often contaminate the brushes, curry combs etc. and so are a potential threat to other horses in the group. Finally, many skin conditions, but not all, cause an irritation. The horse tries to relieve this by rubbing on the stable walls, fence posts, other horses etc. and this assists both in making the condition worse due to self-inflicted damage and in spreading the problem.

DERMATOPHILUS INFECTIONS
Infections with a bacterium called Dermatophilus congolensis are common in both horses and donkeys. It is not generally realized that two distinct conditions, namely Rain Scald and Mud Fever (also called 'grease'), are both caused by this organism. Dermatophilus attacks the surface layer of the skin, leaving it raw and oozing.

Rain scald occurs over the dorsal part of the horse's body i.e. his back. As its name implies it occurs in damp conditions, especially when there is a combination of high temperature and high humidity. For this reason it is commoner in Britain during the warm summer months rather than during the wetter winter months, especially where animals congregate under dripping trees.

The infection causes small areas of skin to ooze, and the resulting fluid dries and mats the hairs together, resulting in a characteristic 'paint brush' effect. As the rain and sweat run over the body the infection is spread, so that the infection is worst over places such as the shoulders and rump where the rain 'runs off'.

Mud fever is an infection of the lower limbs, usually affecting the skin up the back of the pasterns. As its name implies it is commonest in muddy conditions where frequent soaking and knocking of the skin leaves it open to infection. Unlike rain scald, mud fever is not so temperature-dependent. In some countries it occurs most commonly in the winter, when mud and the chapping effects of the cold lower the skin's natural defences. In other parts of the world it is commonest during the spring and summer when the horses are standing for long periods in lush pasture wet with dew or rain. The resultant cracks in bad cases can open up an entry for serious and even fatal infections.

Treatment for all dermatophilus infections is basically the same. The most important step is to keep the affected area dry. With rain scald this will often mean stabling the horse. In the case of mud fever it may be necessary to change the exercising routine or find a new paddock, so that the legs do not get wet. I cannot stress this point too much. If affected areas get wet at all they must be completely dried, if necessary using a hair dryer.

The second step of treatment is to remove any scabs present, which must include clipping off all the hair covering the area, and to keep the affected areas free from scabs. The reason for this is that the scabs protect the surface of the skin where the bacteria are active. It is as if the bacteria live in a layer of moisture between the scab and the skin. If the scabs are removed, the skin tends to dry out and the bacteria can no longer survive. In the initial stages of the infection these scabs may need removing several times a day. You will find that the skin looks inflamed under the scabs, indeed it looks worse after you have finished than it did before you started, but do not be put off by this.

To all intents and purposes you have at this stage completed the treatment, by removing the specialized environment so necessary to the dermatophilus bacteria. Practically any mild antiseptic solution will kill off the remaining exposed bacteria. 1% potash alum or 0.5% copper sulphate solutions are both effective. Antibiotics such as penicillin, either given by injection or applied as a cream, are usually only necessary in severe cases. It is a waste of money to apply expensive creams if you do not also follow the drying part of the treatment.

Treatment should continue until the infection is completely overcome. The presence of even one scab can result in the infection multiplying again. In the case of mud fever it may be worth applying a waterproof barrier cream to the pastern before exercising or exposing the legs to damp conditions during the period after an outbreak of infection.

RINGWORM

Ringworm in horses is caused by one or more of several fungi. When the fungus manages to establish itself on the surface of the skin and around the base of the actual hairs, it releases spores which can spread the infection. Therefore, it is obviously important that grooming equipment, riding tack, rugs or indeed stables and fences of paddocks belonging to infected horses are not used for non-infected horses or cattle. The name ringworm stems from the fact that the affected hairs break off at their bases, leaving a crusty bald patch of skin which is often (but not always) circular in shape. The infection can affect any part of the body, although it is commonest in places where tack etc. rubs the skin. Without treatment affected horses remain

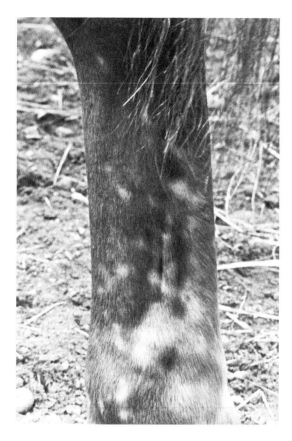

Ringworm on a hind leg.

infected for long periods, and spores on equipment etc. can remain infective for many months.

There are many 'folk remedies' for ringworm, most of them seeking to smother the infection and prevent the spread of any more spores. Only comparatively recently, however, have drugs been available which will reliably kill the fungus. There are two main ways of treating the disease, and they can be used either independently or in combination. Feeding the antibiotic griseofulvin to the horse every day for seven days will kill off the fungus throughout the body. There are also many topical treatments available, but generally only antibiotics such as natamycin actually kill off the fungus when applied to the skin surface. In the USA, of the topical treatments, captan is considered effective on both horse and surroundings.

Other skin problems

SWEET ITCH

Unlike the skin diseases already discussed, sweet itch is not an infection which can spread from horse to horse. Nor, despite what many horse owners think, is it caused by faulty diet or overheating of the blood (whatever that might mean). It is an allergic dermatitis stimulated by the saliva of biting insects. The parts of the body affected may vary from country to country depending on which insect is involved. In Britain the Culicoides midge is responsible, and it is a common cause in the USA. The insects attack the upper midline especially near the mane and tail of the horse. The midge is at its most active during the first two or three hours of daylight and during the last couple of hours of the evening. They are more active when there is high humidity but little wind.

Once a horse or pony has become allergic to insect bites it will always remain so. The allergic response is so irritating that such horses will rub the affected areas until they are raw and hairless. There can be few more sorry sights than a sweet-itch pony with only the bare remnants of a mane and tail, rubbing already raw patches of skin. Once the hairs of the mane and tail have been lost in this way it will take many months before they regrow to their normal length.

Treatment must concentrate on preventing access for the insect responsible. Affected horses should be stabled, especially when the biting insect is active. For Culicoides this means that it is safe for affected horses to graze during the heat of the day but not in the morning and evening. Other flies may worry the horse during this grazing period, but they will not aggravate the course of the sweet itch. The Culicoides midge is most active in the months of May, June and September, so these are the times of peak incidence of this condition. Fly repellants, especially the new synthetic pyrethroids (pyrethrins in USA), can be a great help in preventing sweet itch. Unfortunately they have to be applied to both horse and stable at weekly intervals, or other frequent intervals, if they are to be effective. Anti-inflammatory drugs, principally the long-acting corticosteroids, can help to alleviate the symptoms but they are no substitute for preventing the fly bites in the first place.

NODULAR SKIN DISEASES

Horses may suddenly develop small nodules (ranging in size from 1 mm–1.5 cm or $\frac{1}{26}$ in–$\frac{5}{8}$ in diameter) in their skin. These nodules are commonest over the saddle area and the chest wall, although they may also spread forward to the neck. The cause of the condition is unknown, although microscopic examination of skin samples suggests that some form of allergic response, or collagen damage, is involved.

Sweet itch at an early stage, on a pony's mane. Arrows indicate raw patches where rubbing has caused thickening of the skin.

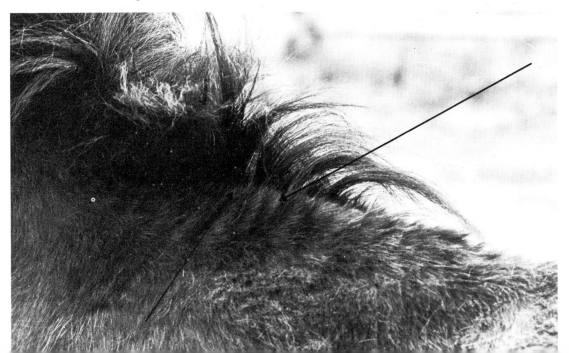

Chestnuts and bays are more commonly affected than other coat colours; and soft, fine-skinned horses are more commonly affected than coarser-skinned animals.

Over the course of several days the nodules appear to come to a 'head' and gain a small scab. If the damaged collagen 'plug' falls out, the horses then recover spontaneously. Unfortunately there is little available in Britain in the way of a permanent cure for those horses where the nodules remain; in the USA, 'coring' the nodules with a special needle is quite effective. Once the dead collagen is gone the nodule subsides. Corticosteroids may give a temporary improvement but often the nodules return when treatment is stopped. If only a few nodules are present, surgical removal may be the answer. This is especially the case when the nodules are on the saddle area, where pressure may cause them to ulcerate. In badly affected animals it may be worth trying to establish whether a food allergy is involved, and adjusting the diet accordingly.

WARBLES

The skin nodules I have just described should be differentiated from warbles, which may also affect the saddle area. Warble fly larvae can migrate through the horse from the legs, where the adult fly lays its eggs, up to the back. Here, instead of 'the adult flies' emerging through the skin as they do in cattle, they encyst and form a permanent swelling in the skin.

Initially these swellings are painful but eventually many of them settle down, just leaving a painless blemish. When the saddle area is involved surgical removal of the larva and its surrounding cyst may well be necessary.

HABRONEMIASIS ('SUMMER SORE' IN USA)

The stomach worm Habronema is found in many tropical and hot climates. The eggs or larvae of this worm may infest flies which land on or live in the pasture. When these infested flies land on a horse's wound the habronema larvae emerge and burrow into the animal's skin. The irritation they cause gives rise to a raw, swollen area of skin. This condition has been very difficult indeed to control, but a new class of anthelmintics called the ivermectins shows every sign of curing the problem.

LICE

Horse lice are small yellowish-brown creatures, 2–3 mm ($\frac{1}{12}$ – $\frac{1}{8}$ in) in length. They live on the surface of the skin, mainly over the neck and shoulder area. It is thought that the intense itching seen in affected horses is caused by both the movement of the lice and by the biting which occurs when they feed. As a result large bald patches of skin are formed.

Lice spend their whole life on the horse. Spreading from horse to horse usually occurs when they rub up against each other, although grooming equipment can also spread the infestation. Unusually the louse life cycle can only be completed at low temperatures, so this is a problem only seen during the winter months. Hardly any adult lice survive the summer temperatures, although their eggs obviously do survive ready to hatch out the following winter. As it only takes about ten days from egg to adult louse, the parasites can increase in numbers very quickly once they become established in a horse's coat.

There are a wide variety of louse powders and anti-parasitic shampoos available. In Britain the commonest drug incorporated is gamma Benzene Hexa-Chloride (B.H.C.). In severe infestations it may be necessary to clip away all the thick winter coat and burn it, leaving the skin itself exposed to whichever drug is being used.

WARTS

Warts are a form of skin tumour, caused by a virus. It follows that warts can spread from animal to animal. Young horses often develop large numbers of warts around their muzzles, and once one horse in the group has become affected other horses often 'catch' the same condition. Most warts disappear eventually on their own, often as quickly as they appeared.

Equine sarcoids are a large form of wart, found anywhere over the horse's body. These large growths are often called angleberries. Sarcoids are usually permanent. Even surgery may only remove them temporarily, although freezing or radiation techniques have shown more success.

9 Diseases of the senses

Diseases of the eye

The horse's eye is relatively free from veterinary problems. One reason for this is that the muscles of the eyelids are very powerful and quickly close the lids if there is any danger threatening the eye. It is not possible to test a horse's sight with any accuracy; the most information we can hope for is whether a horse can 'see' and respond to a bright light shining into one of his eyes. The precise control we exert over riding and driving horses means that quite marked damage to the eye may have no apparent effect on performance at all.

EYE INJURIES

The commonest problem affecting horses' eyes is injury. Injury to the eyelids will usually result in the eye being at least partially closed. The sensitive tissues swell rapidly, as anyone who has been punched in the eye will verify, and a greatly increased amount of tears is produced. This fluid will very readily become infected, and it is important in treating such injuries not only to attempt to reduce the inflammation, but also to administer drugs which will prevent any infection becoming established. Combined corticosteroid and antibiotic ophthalmic ointments (never any ointment not made specifically for use in eyes) will often work 'miracles' on swollen, pussy eyelids. In the USA corticosteroids are not favoured for use on eyes and eyelids.

Like most animals the horse has a nictitating membrane, or third eyelid. In human beings this

The structure of the eye.

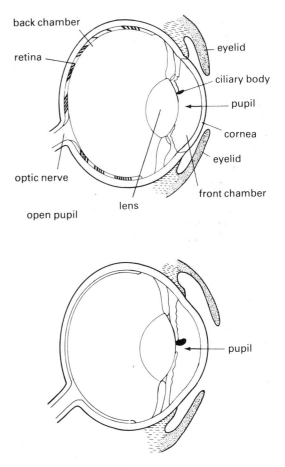

open pupil

closed pupil

is merely a fleshy lump of tissue at the inner corner of the eye, but in horses it is a pink membrane which can be moved from the inner corner right across the surface of the eyeball, without needing to close the eyelids. This membrane is susceptible to injury in the same way that the eyelids are.

Foreign bodies of many kinds have been found in horses' eyes, where they cause an intense irritation. Obviously no amount of medication will cure this problem unless the foreign body itself is removed. In some cases, especially when the thin outer coat, or hull, of cereal grains is involved, it may be impossible for the ordinary horseman to detect the presence of a foreign body in the eye, and examination with an ophthalmoscope may be necessary.

The eyeball itself is very sensitive to injury, especially bruising. It is important that you realise that inflammation of the cornea, as the transparent front covering of the eye is called, shows by a milky opaqueness over the affected area. If the injury has been more severe, especially if it involves breaking the surface of the cornea, red blood vessels may develop and grow across the corneal surface from the outer rim towards the affected area. Although treatment will usually eliminate these symptoms in time the horse may be left with a small 'scar' on the cornea. This permanent blemish will show up on later eye examination, e.g. at the time of sale. Whether the blemish is likely to interfere with the horse's usefulness by interfering with his vision when jumping etc. will obviously depend on the area of cornea involved.

PERIODIC OPHTHALMIA (UVEITIS, IRIDOCYCLITIS IN USA)

Periodic ophthalmia, or moon blindness, is a disease of the horse's eye which occurs throughout the world, especially where the standard of management is poor. The cause is unknown, although both low vitamin B levels in the diet and Leptospirosis infections in the eye are frequently thought to be responsible. Since less than 20% of those affected ever have a second attack, 'periodic' is misleading. In those having a recurrence, the disease comes and goes at irregular intervals. During the periods of apparent recovery, which may last days or years, the eye may appear perfectly normal. In the acute stage the eye is closed and watery. The horse is very sensitive to light, which it tries to avoid. The eyeball itself may appear white due to inflammatory changes inside.

There is no specific treatment for this condition. Where Leptospirosis infection is present, antibiotics may be of value. Unfortunately the end result of periodic ophthalmia is usually blindness. Prevention of the inflammatory changes by dilating the pupil and administering steroids has sometimes been useful in minimizing permanent damage from ophthalmia.

Diseases of the nervous system

Thankfully nervous diseases are rare in the horse. There are some conditions which may appear to involve the nervous system but in fact do not do so. A sudden paralysis of the hindquarters seen in horses during galloping, for instance, has been shown to be due to the blocking off of the blood supply to the limbs rather than any fault in the nerves themselves.

On the other hand, head shaking in horses is a condition which, in the absence of any other obvious cause, such as teeth problems or sinusitis, it is thought must be due to some fault in the nervous system, even though it has not proved possible to find out what that fault might be. A 'head shaker' is a horse which shakes his head up and down so violently when exercised that the horse often becomes unrideable. The onset of the condition is often very sudden, but once it has occurred it is usually a permanent problem. In Britain head shaking only occurs during the summer months and affected horses will perform completely normally during the colder weather. Literally hundreds of causes have been considered for the condition. When a horse first starts to shake his head most owners are convinced that flies are involved in some way because the shaking is worse in situations of warmth and humidity where flies congregate.

WOBBLER DISEASE

Wobbler disease is a progressive nervous disease of horses. Although it first appears in young horses, under two years of age, the condition always becomes more and more severe. At first the horse appears to be slightly wobbly and uncertain on his hind legs. In some horses the disease may progress so far that eventually the horse is either completely paralysed in his hindquarters or is even unable to control his forelegs properly. Making the horse walk backwards or in a tight circle usually makes the incoordination more obvious.

Interestingly, there appear to be several distinct differences between wobblers in Britain and those seen in America. In America the condition is more common in male horses, whereas in Britain this distinction is not so obvious. The cause of the nervous symptoms is pressure on the spinal cord due to a narrowing of the spinal canal. The site along the horse's neck where this occurs also appears to differ between the two countries. Although surgical relief of the narrowing in the bony canal has been attempted, and achieved, the condition usually goes uncured.

RADIAL PARALYSIS

The radial nerve is the main nerve to the fore leg. In the shoulder region this nerve lies comparatively unprotected near the point of the shoulder. If a horse receives a blow or knock to this region the nerve may well be damaged. The importance of this is that the affected leg then dangles limply, and at first glance it might be thought that the leg is broken. Providing that the nerve is only bruised, and not permanently damaged, the paralysis will, in time, disappear and the leg return to normal.

GRASS SICKNESS

Grass sickness is a disease of the alimentary tract which is due to damage to the nerves supplying the various internal organs. At present the cause of the disease is unknown, although the damage which is sustained by the nervous system has been well documented. It would appear that the cause is 'infectious', because taking samples from an infected horse and injecting them into another horse has been shown to produce the disease.

Grass sickness is usually a fatal disease. In acute cases the horse can die within 48 hours, but in chronic cases it may take weeks or months before the horse dies. The disease causes a form of paralysis of the stomach wall, and the stomach becomes swollen with a green liquid. The horse also becomes unable to swallow, and this is often the first symptom seen by the horse owner. The horse just plays with his food and water, but he cannot swallow any of it. The horse's intestines, on the other hand, become overactive, and except in acute cases he may well develop diarrhoea.

There is no cure for grass sickness. Euthanasia is nearly always necessary to spare the horse the severe pain which the swollen stomach causes.

10 A note on the future; and the old horse

I hope that by this stage you will be aware of some of the great advances in veterinary knowledge which have so transformed our attitudes to many horse ailments during the last quarter of a century. Science, however, is never static, and veterinary science shows no signs of resting on its laurels on existing knowledge.

Veterinary research is carried out on two main fronts. Much of the research into new drugs is carried out by, or in association with, the pharmaceutical companies. Drugs such as prostaglandins to control the mare's oestrus cycle or the bronchodilator clenbuterol are examples of this development. Development and final marketing of such research products depends on the company anticipating a market for the drug. It is not sufficient to discover an effective drug, it must be economically viable. It follows that pharmaceutical research tends to be directed at ailments affecting large numbers of horses and ponies, rather than just the specialist élite.

Research into surgical and diagnostic techniques tends, on the other hand, to be carried out in university departments and specialist research institutes. Initially these techniques are often carried out on only the most expensive horses. This is because the high economic cost can only be justified to the owner of a high value horse. In most cases, however, as the techniques become more widely used they 'filter down' the pyramid of horses until they are being applied to quite ordinary horses and ponies. Endoscopy, used to investigate the horse's respiratory system, is an example of a technique which is fast spreading out of the academic world into general veterinary practice.

No mention of veterinary research would be complete without acknowledging the great debt we owe to human medicine. Many of our drugs and techniques have, over the years, been borrowed from our medical colleagues. It isn't always that way round, I am glad to say. Warfarin therapy in navicular disease is an example of where we have shown the medical world a solution to a problem which has its counterpart in the human species.

The old horse

Unfortunately the only certainty in the future is that sooner or later all living creatures must die, including our beloved horses. In many cases nature takes its course and we just find the horse has died peacefully. In other cases the horse becomes too old or infirm to work and we are faced with a dilemma over what action, if any, we should take.

In parts of the world where significant amounts of horseflesh are eaten then the majority of such old horses are killed for meat. This can be done quickly and painlessly, without any suffering to the horse. If the presence of some form of disease renders the horse unsuitable for human consumption, then in Britain the knackerman or the hunt kennels will perform the same service.

Painful though it is to consider such matters there are occasions when a veterinary surgeon (veterinarian) is glad to have the option available to him of putting an end to a horse's suffering. It is, after all, not an option which is ever legally available to our medical colleagues, no matter how distressing the circumstances. The veterinary surgeon (veterinarian) may shoot the horse through the skull, which kills the animal instantly, even though reflex muscle movements may be seen for some minutes afterwards. Alternatively he may inject an enormous overdose of barbiturate directly into the horse's bloodstream through the jugular vein. In this case the horse collapses as if anaesthetized but instead dies within seconds. Obviously if barbiturates are used for euthanasia the carcase has no commercial value.

I would not like to close this book on an unhappy note. The whole aim of the book has, after all, been to help you to treat and prevent ailments which might cause suffering in your horse. Although any horse aged over fifteen or twenty must be classified as old, providing you stick rigidly to a good management regime and do not ask for a higher level of 'performance' than his physical capabilities allow, you can enjoy watching your horse's 'old age' as much as he enjoys living it.

The horse is said to be very intelligent, and to be a good learner. It is, perhaps, unfortunate that he learns bad habits as quickly as good ones, but no horse is really perfect (except in the 'For Sale' advertisements). We have one advantage over the horse's intelligence, though. We can ask for advice and benefit from it. Hopefully some of the advice within this book will have been of value to you. It is not possible, however, to cover every topic in one volume; if you are uncertain about any aspect of your horse's health, seek professional advice. Your horse will thank you for doing so.

A physiotherapy machine in use, a modern technique for treating horses.

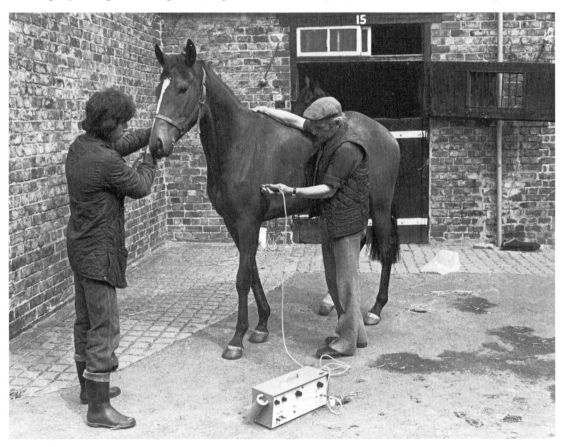

Glossary

Anthelmintics Drugs which kill or remove parasitic worms which live inside the horse.

Blood salts (electrolytes) Chemical substances such as sodium, potassium, chloride etc which are present in the blood both as a means of circulating them round the body and as a chemical force which maintains the balance of fluids within the body.

Bronchodilator A chemical which specifically relaxes the muscles in the walls of the air tubes or bronchioles in the lung. This increases the airway.

Bronchospasm The contraction of the muscles in the walls of the bronchioles in the lung. This decreases the size of the airway.

Concussion (percussion) The vibratory shock which travels through the affected part of the body, eg when the horse's foot hits the ground.

Cycle Because the mare shows a regular pattern of sexual activity, the period from the start of one oestrus period through to the start of the next (usually 21 days) is often called the oestrus cycle.

Echography A system where an ultra-sound source sends out directional impulses through the body tissues. The echoes received are transformed into an X-ray type image on a viewing screen.

Electrolytes see **Blood salts**

Endoscopy Using a narrow tube (originally rigid but now usually flexible) which combines a powerful light source with viewing lenses in order to see inside the body. Used mainly in the horse for examining the respiratory system.

Enzymes Chemical substances which have the ability to change one chemical into another.

Euthanasia Causing the painless death of an animal. This is often preferable to leaving the horse suffering, eg with a badly broken leg.

Faeces The waste solids which a horse must excrete via the rectum.

Glanders A bacterial respiratory infection of horses.

Glycogen A form of starch which the horse manufactures in its muscles as a store of energy for future use.

In foal A pregnant mare is said to be 'in foal'.

Lactic acid A breakdown product formed when the horse uses his glycogen reserves to provide energy.

Larynx A rigid chamber at the top of the trachea or wind-pipe. Because it contains the vocal chords, it is sometimes called the voice-box.

Membranes The thin flexible covering to internal surfaces inside the body, eg the lining of the stomach or the walls of the trachea (wind-pipe).

Nebuliser A machine which manufactures a vapour containing minute droplets of a liquid such as a drug.

Nictitating membrane The so-called 'third eyelid' which is present at the inner corner of the eye.

Oesophagus The flexible tube which joins the mouth to the stomach.

Oestrus The period when a mare is sexually

active and will accept mating with a stallion.

Pharynx The chamber inside the horse's head where the mouth, larynx, oesophagus and nasal passages all inter-connect.

Progesterone A female sex hormone which inhibits sexual activity, and is thus present during pregnancy and between oestrus periods.

Prosthesis An artificial replacement for a damaged part of the body.

Respiratory system The nasal passages, pharynx, larynx, trachea and lungs together make up the respiratory system.

Salivary salts Chemicals found in the liquid saliva which is mixed with food during the process of chewing.

Selenium One of a number of chemical elements which are essential to the body but are only needed in minute amounts, and are therefore called 'trace elements'.

Sound A sound horse is one which does not have any illness or defect present which is at the moment or which might in the future, affect his usefulness. Sometimes used in a limited sense to mean a horse which is not lame.

Suture A stitch used to join cut or damaged parts of the body.

Ultra-sound A very high frequency sound-wave used for diagnostic purposes.

Unsound An unsound horse has some defect present which either is now, or might in the future, affect his usefulness. Sometimes used in a more limited sense to mean a lame horse.

Index